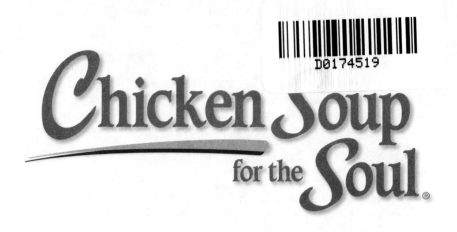

Living
with Alzheimer's
& Other Dementias

Chicken Soup for the Soul: Living with Alzheimer's & Other Dementias
101 Stories of Caregiving, Coping, and Compassion
Amy Newmark, Angela Timashenka Geiger
Published by Chicken Soup for the Soul Publishing, LLC www.chickensoup.com

The publisher gratefully acknowledges the many publishers and individuals, including
the Alzheimer's Association, who granted Chicken Soup for the Soul permission to
reprint the cited material.

Front cover photo courtesy of iStockPhoto.com/AleksandarNakic (©AleksandarNakic).
Interior photo courtesy of iStockPhoto.com/UmbertoPantalone (©UmbertoPantalone).

Cover and Interior Design & Layout by Brian Taylor, Pneuma Books, LLC

Distributed to the booktrade by Simon & Schuster. SAN: 200-2442

Publisher's Cataloging-in-Publication Data
(Prepared by The Donohue Group)

Chicken soup for the soul : living with Alzheimer's & other dementias :
  101 stories of caregiving, coping, and compassion / [compiled by] Amy
  Newmark [and] Angela Timashenka Geiger.

    pages ; cm

  A joint project with the Alzheimer's Association.
  ISBN: 978-1-61159-934-3

    1. Alzheimer's disease--Patients--Care--Literary collections. 2. Alzheimer's disease-
  -Patients--Care--Anecdotes. 3. Dementia--Patients--Care--Literary collections. 4.
  Dementia--Patients--Care--Anecdotes. 5. Anecdotes. I. Newmark, Amy, compiler.
  II. Geiger, Angela Timashenka, compiler. III. Title: Living with Alzheimer's & other
  dementias : 101 stories of caregiving, coping, and compassion IV. Title: Living with
  Alzheimer's and other dementias : 101 stories of caregiving, coping, and compassion

PN6071.D46 C45 2014
810.8/02/0356/1   2014930199

PRINTED IN THE UNITED STATES OF AMERICA
on acid∞free paper

24 23 22 21 20 19 18 17 16 15 14   01 02 03 04 05 06 07 08 09 10 11

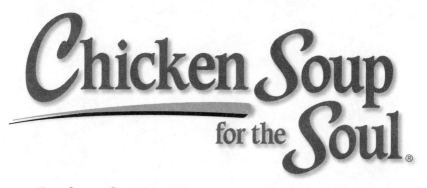

Living
with Alzheimer's
& Other Dementias

101 Stories of Caregiving,
Coping, and Compassion

Amy Newmark
Angela Timashenka Geiger

Chicken Soup for the Soul Publishing, LLC
Cos Cob, CT

Contents

❸
~Strategies and Tips for Coping~

❹
~Next Steps and Tough Choices~

❺
~Taking the Journey with Your Parent~

❻
~Younger-Onset Alzheimer's~

❼
~In Sickness and In Health~

8

~The Lighter Side~

9

~New Ways to Make Connections~

10

~It Takes a Village~

⓫

~The Special Bond with Grandchildren~

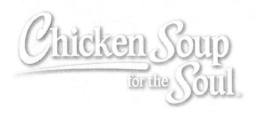

Introduction

Stories can conquer fear, you know. They can make the heart bigger.
~Ben Okri

Alzheimer's disease was first discovered in 1906, and in more than 100 years, a lot has changed. For too long, those facing the disease struggled in silence. Consequently, the misconceptions, misdiagnoses, myths, and stigmas around Alzheimer's grew and grew, partially due to our own inability to find the words to share our experiences.

The stories inside this book reveal a new world for the Alzheimer's community—a world where we've discovered the strength to speak up and work together to defeat Alzheimer's disease and other dementias. This new world is one that the Alzheimer's Association®, the leader in Alzheimer's care, support and research, is proud to help grow and shape. More and more, Alzheimer's is discussed among friends and family in the home, in workplaces, in places of worship, and beyond. People with Alzheimer's participate in support groups and online forums and advocate for needed change. It is no longer assumed that Alzheimer's is a normal part of aging—instead, it's recognized as a fatal disease that demands better methods of diagnosis and treatment.

Indeed, the dialogue is increasing, but we still have a long way to go. Currently, at least 44 million people worldwide are living with Alzheimer's or another dementia, and if trends continue, this number could triple by 2050 to 115 million. As the baby boom generation ages, Alzheimer's will continue to escalate, threatening families, communities, and nations with economic, physical, and emotional devastation.

That's why it's so important that this collection of stories exists—so that while we press forward with care and support for affected families, and strive to advance research that will one day lead to a cure, we're sharing information, compassion, and advice with one another. We're speaking up about the realities of Alzheimer's, and together, we're breaking through the stigmas that exist.

Receiving an Alzheimer's diagnosis—or learning that a friend or family member has the disease—is often a shock. In Chapter 1, "Accepting a New Reality," our authors relate how they adjusted to life with Alzheimer's. Ginny Dubose, who works in the senior housing industry, encourages people to "join the journey" and live in the moment alongside the person with dementia. Singer Joey McIntyre of New Kids on the Block describes how he acknowledges his mom's sense of self, which is still strong despite her battle with Alzheimer's.

In the second chapter, "What Does It Feel Like?", some extremely brave authors living with dementia attempt to answer this all-too-common—and perplexing—question. These individuals express their intimate thoughts about the disease while describing the ways in which they work to live their best life. While their perspectives are unique, these courageous contributors share a sentiment aptly stated by Cynthia A. Guzman: "As this disease progresses, I won't remember anyone, but I want to live my life so that people will remember me."

Those impacted by Alzheimer's know that coping strategies are critical to moving forward after a diagnosis. Chapter 3, "Strategies and Tips for Coping," features insightful and useful tactics for life with the disease. Fred Kinsinger writes about how he created a special clock for his wife, one with only an hour hand—a gift that solves a practical challenge while also serving as a symbol of his love. Johanna Richardson tells us how she "learned to lie" in order to be a better caregiver, and Laura Suihkonen Jones encourages those affected to build a fellowship with others facing the disease.

As Alzheimer's inevitably progresses, people facing the disease are confronted with difficult questions: How do I deal with what's happening right now? How do I prepare for the future? In Chapter 4, "Next Steps and Tough Choices," authors share how they tackled issues about home care, assisted living facilities, driving, and other challenges—and how they dealt with the conflicting emotions that came along with them. After moving her mother into a nursing home, Carolyn Mers tells us, "Did I have doubts about my decision? Almost every day. Did I think I could do a better job? Sometimes. Did I know that she was in a good place? Always." The honesty of these authors will provide strength to anyone who has faced a similar situation.

Alzheimer's disease often creates a heartbreaking role reversal: Spouses assume the other's responsibilities, grandchildren "watch" their grandparents, and perhaps most difficult of all, children must care for their parents. Chapter 5, "Taking the Journey with Your Parent," provides inspiration and coping techniques from those who've been there. But this experience, however painful, is not without its own reward, as Ann Napoletan relates. Describing her relationship with her mother after Alzheimer's, Ann says, "Ultimately… our connection was strengthened exponentially, and I felt closer to her than ever before. It's a testament to the fact that even immense loss and heartbreak can bring blessings."

Our "Younger-Onset Alzheimer's" chapter offers inspiration and support from a unique perspective. Currently, there are more than 200,000 people under the age of sixty-five living with Alzheimer's; these individuals and their caregivers face a unique set of challenges at work and home. In "The Hardest Day," Karen M. Henley describes her husband's diagnosis at age thirty-six, his brave fight with the disease, and the pride she feels that her two young children, Courtney and Brandon, helped care for their father at home until his passing.

Marriage vows, and the ways in which they're tested by Alzheimer's, bring new light to their meaning. Chapter 7, "In Sickness and In Health," details how the disease can change and deepen the relationship between spouses. Deborah Shouse learns a valuable lesson from her once-stoic father as he openly revels in her mother's spirit and beauty, even as he loses her to Alzheimer's: "I fully understood what my father had always known: Beauty is there, if you're looking with your heart."

While Alzheimer's causes immeasurable pain, the disease also presents us with moments of laughter we learn to appreciate in order to get through the tough days. Chapter 8, "The Lighter Side," includes some hilarious anecdotes from authors like Jean Salisbury Campbell, who tells a laugh-out-loud story about her mother's insistence that a bird was loose in the house—and, when revealed to be true, what happens when the family cat finds it. This chapter demonstrates the power of laughter and the valuable lessons that can come with a smile.

Many of this book's contributors share their experiences with art, music, dance, and other forms of therapy as a way to reach the person living with the disease. Our "New Ways to Make Connections" chapter describes how undiscovered abilities and long-ago melodies can spark moments of clarity and connection. In Robert Nussbaum's story, "The Man in My Mother's Room," the sounds of Frank Sinatra bring his mother back to him, if only for a few minutes. In "Hidden Talents" Marjorie Hilkert connects with her father as he demonstrates his previously unknown gift for painting.

Alzheimer's is a disease that no one can face alone. We draw strength from our family, friends, and sometimes even strangers—people who are walking the same path alongside us. In Chapter 10, "It Takes a Village," authors convey stories of unexpected friendship and compassion. Louise Harris Berlin recounts how her brothers, Russ and Reed, embraced everyone in their dad's memory care unit, making the entire group a new kind of family, and even continuing to visit the other residents after their father was gone.

We close the book with Chapter 11, "The Special Bond with Grandchildren," highlighting this powerful relationship, which Alzheimer's often heightens. Grandchildren learn how to be caregivers, take on responsibilities far beyond their years, and learn to value every moment with their grandparents. In "Understanding Nana," actress Sarah Rafferty recounts the fierce protectiveness she felt as her grandmother battled Alzheimer's, and the ways in which Nana will live on through the future generations of their family.

Anyone affected by Alzheimer's or another dementia should feel a sense of ownership when they pick up this book. I hope that in these stories, you can see yourself, you can learn something, and that you are proud of this movement—of this caring and compassionate community—that you've helped build. I urge you to take action in the fight, whether by sharing your experience, speaking up, or spreading the word—so that someday, the only story we have left to write is about the end of Alzheimer's disease.

~Angela Timashenka Geiger
Chief Strategy Officer, Alzheimer's Association

Travel with the person to where he or she is in time. If the person's memory is focused on a particular time in his or her life, engage in conversation about recollections with an understanding that this is his or her current reality.

"How to respond"
alz.org/care

Living with Alzheimer's

Chapter 1

& Other Dementias

Accepting a New Reality

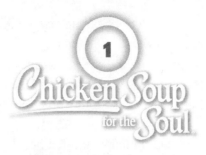

My Mom
the Fighter Pilot

We can do no great things, only small things with great love.
~Mother Teresa

A few years after Mom was diagnosed with Alzheimer's she started to believe what her mind was telling her. A few Alzheimer's caregiver seminars had taught me not to question her imagination, so that made it easier for me to just listen and accept it when one summer day Mom said she was a fighter pilot in the Air Force.

We were at Mom's favorite diner. She was well liked there because she always kissed the manager and all the waiters, but I noticed Mom was not her happy self that day. She just wanted to go straight to our usual table and stare out the window, gazing up at the sky. It was a perfect blue-sky day, with cotton ball clouds.

"What are you thinking about, Mom?" I asked. That's when she told me she was once a fighter pilot in the Air Force and that one of her missions was to rescue all the children from the war. As Mom was saying this, tears rolled down her face and she told me she had jumped from the plane to rescue the children, but she was not able to rescue them all, because she could only take as many as she could carry. She cried when she said she had to leave some children behind.

I looked at her and said, "Mom, you did the best you could, it was better to save some than not saving any at all." I'm not sure she was listening; I could only hope it helped.

Then one day Mom told me she got a call from the military telling her she was going to receive the highest Medal of Honor for rescuing those children. For weeks Mom would tell me she got another call, and another.

I decided to buy her a medal, and tell her the military had contacted me and was sending me her Medal of Honor, to be presented to her on her upcoming birthday. My daughter said she wanted to make up a Certificate of Honor, so she could give it to her grandmother with the Medal of Honor.

Mom was getting worse by the month now, and I had a feeling this might be the last birthday where she would be able to communicate very well. I knew I needed to make this birthday extra special, and the one thing Mom loved to do was dance. I decided to take Mom, Dad, my daughter, her husband, and my partner to a Latin American restaurant that had a band.

When I told Mom where I was taking her for her birthday, she was so excited she told me she wanted to wear something red. My older sister, who is in the military and was away, sent her a beautiful red silk blouse, and I took Mom to the salon.

When we all got to the restaurant, Mom was so excited she was smiling from ear to ear. I ordered Mom her favorite drink, sangria, and as soon as the band began to play, my daughter took her to the dance floor for her first birthday dance. After that Mom danced with me, with my partner, and with anyone who wanted to dance with her. She was on a roll, having the time of her life.

Then it was time for the cake. We all stood up when it came, and my daughter read Mom the Certificate of Honor, and I presented her with the Medal of Honor. Everyone in the restaurant stood up and applauded, congratulating Mom. Mom was so surprised and so happy that she got up and kissed every single person in that restaurant.

It's been a year now and Mom is unable to talk or walk on her own, but I am so thankful we took her dancing for her birthday and presented her with her Medal of Honor.

~Doris Leddy

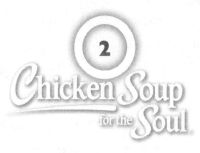

Join the Journey

When we are no longer able to change a situation,
we are challenged to change ourselves.
~Victor Frankl

I work in senior housing—a safe, friendly, comfortable community for seniors that provides them with an opportunity to live independently or with some assistance while still maintaining their sense of self-worth and independence. I have done this work for more than twenty years, and many times have heard family members say, "I don't know how you people do it! I can't deal with just one elderly parent, and here you all are having to work day in and day out with so many of them!"

Here's my answer: We join the journey. We love them and care for them just the way they are now. They are brand new to us. Because we have no history with Aunt Mae or Grandpa Joe, we aren't disappointed by their need to use incontinence products, or their inability to remember their address, or even their constant questions about what day it is.

We love and care for the people they have become. There's no past history for us. No memories of how they built their own company from the ground up, or helped raise funds for the Sunday school wing of their church, or organized the neighborhood carpools. We love them today—incontinent, feisty, forgetful.

We join their journey, and we know lots of ways to help them help themselves when family members get frustrated. Almost everyone grows up seeing their parent or grandparent as strong and capable, but when that former math professor can no longer remember how to write a check, families can get embarrassed—not for themselves, but for the parent who used to be. It's okay with us. It's our job, and more importantly, it's our calling to love and respect the person that math professor is today—not to try to steer him down a path he no longer sees or understands.

Once, one of our residents became agitated during an afternoon cloudburst. Daughter Carol was trying to reason with her mom, who was standing in the hallway, wearing her raincoat and looking for an umbrella so she could go outside. Miss Caroline, a normally gracious woman, but a woman with Alzheimer's, had not been outside of our building unaccompanied in quite some time. She had never, as far as I knew, become upset because of rainy weather and we were all—her daughter, her assigned caregiver, and I—at a loss as to how to calm her and encourage her to stay indoors. Finally, after about ten minutes of trying to talk her out of going outside, someone asked her a question she could grasp and answer:

"Miss Caroline, why do you need to go out in this awful rain?" This mother of eight sons and one daughter gave a deep sigh and looked each of us in the face as she answered: "The children will be coming home from school. I don't want them to get wet—I have to meet them at the bus stop."

This was a Join the Journey moment. A light dawned for us all—including the grown daughter who was standing right there. We quickly assured her that a neighbor was picking up the children and that she would bring them home. Satisfied that her children were safe and dry, Miss Caroline returned to her apartment, took off her raincoat, and settled in her room for the rest of the afternoon.

Join the Journey. It's hard. So very hard—especially for those who remember when their loved ones were titans of business, supervisors of factories, the go-to moms for bake sales and carpools.

But to live in their moment, to allow them to have the pleasure of the day without forcing a reality they no longer understand—now that is love at its finest.

It's not easy. And not everyone is a Miss Caroline, willing to hear your words and absorb them and accept them. But many are.

Join the Journey. Let go of their past, and your own, and spend whatever time is left to your loved one on their terms. Don't take their loss of memory personally. Those memories you shared from your childhood are still precious to them. They're just locked away. They aren't deliberately forgetting their keys... their glasses... their teeth. Those things just aren't important to them the way they are to you and me.

Join the Journey. Love them for who they are in this moment. Be old enough, wise enough, and caring enough to set yourself aside. Take heart that the parent who raised you, the grandmother who baked you cookies, the father who taught you to fish is still in there and still needs your care, your love, your patience. Though you may be a stranger to them, they can still recognize kindness.

It's not easy loving someone with Alzheimer's or other forms of dementia. But it's oh so important that you do, and it's a lot easier when you love the new person they've become and join them on their journey.

~Ginny Dubose

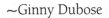

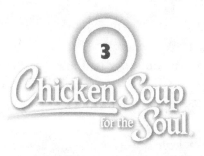

The Little Woman

The only rock I know that stays steady,
the only institution I know that works
is the family.
~Lee Iacocca

"Mom, is anything wrong?" My grandmother didn't answer. My dad gently took her hands in his and asked once more. "Mom, what's wrong?"

"Let me try," my mom said quietly. "Mother, can you hear me?" She reached for my grandmother's hands, but the second she touched them my grandmother brushed her away.

Even though my grandmother had dementia, she had been able to converse with people, although most of the time her words made little sense. But lately, my grandmother seemed indignant and reserved. As my parents searched for an answer, they had noticed that when Dad visited alone, Grandma would speak. Yet when Mom visited, Grandma seemed agitated.

The following week my parents arrived together. Dad slid Grandma's lunch tray in front of her, but my grandmother shoved it away.

"How dare you bring your little woman on our lunch date!" My grandmother glared at my mom, who looked completely devastated.

"What do you mean, Mom?" Dad asked patiently. "This is my wife, your daughter-in-law, don't you remember?"

"And you, little woman, how dare you come here with my

husband!" With those words my grandmother flung her lunch on the floor.

Long ago my grandmother had affectionately called my mom "little woman" because she was tiny, unlike Grandma, who was tall and big-framed. Perhaps she remembered the name, but had forgotten my mom.

It might have been funny, but Grandma had accused her of being the other woman. During the next visit, Mom tried enticing Grandma with a box of her favorite chocolates, but she refused to acknowledge her.

When my father told the staff what had happened they explained that some women with dementia, like my grandmother, become confused and believe their sons are their husbands. The staff suggested we allow a week to pass before my mom visited again.

Even though my parents kept a good sense of humor during this period, I know it disheartened Mom. She had always been close to my grandmother and now she couldn't visit her.

As the years passed, Grandma became silent, even with my dad. However the sight of my mom still disturbed her, so Mom and Dad gave up. Then one day the phone rang. It was the nursing home.

"We're sorry, but her body is shutting down. We thought you'd want to know so that you can call the family together to say goodbye."

Almost thirteen difficult years had passed. While my dad handled every emergency that concerned my grandmother, my mom had stood by helplessly. She yearned to see my grandmother one last time. She needed to express her love and say goodbye, even if it meant Grandma might become hostile.

As my mother approached the room she could see my grandmother on the bed. She had her eyes closed and each breath she took was slow and shallow.

"Mom? It's me, Mom," she whispered, "the little woman." She reached out and gently touched my grandmother's hand. She worried that Grandma might throw a fit, but instead my grandmother clasped my mother's hand tightly and squeezed it.

With a smile on her face, Mom reminisced about old times and updated my grandmother on the lives of her grandchildren. While she chuckled through some stories, she cried through others. Then she told Grandma how much everyone loved her and how much she would be missed.

Most of all, she thanked her for being such a wonderful mother and grandmother. My grandma held her hand the entire time, and though Grandma never said a word, my mother believed she knew and understood everything Mom had told her. These two beautiful women, who loved each other so much, were finally family again.

~Jill Burns

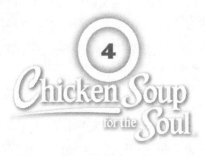

Drama Come to Life

*What happens to the wide-eyed observer when the window between reality
and unreality breaks and the glass begins to fly?*
~Author Unknown

As I stepped in front of the audience, a gentleman in the front row caught my attention. He was immaculately dressed, well groomed, and had a genteel and refined demeanor. He held his head and shoulders erect, and his eyes sparkled. As my performance progressed, I could see he was clearly impressed with each vignette. Occasionally, he would nod or whisper affirmation of the character's lines. It all seemed to touch him deeply. I didn't quite understand why, but there seemed to be something extraordinary happening. Was I witnessing some deep level of hope — or even need?

When performing, I always try to remain aware of how individual members of the audience respond. The nature of that response can be a clear indication as to whether I have gained or lost that vital, dynamic connection required between actor and audience. As an actress and playwright, my aim is always to craft characterizations that reveal the mysteries and emotional complexities of life.

Thus, while observing this particular gentleman's reactions, I was suddenly struck by the thought that he was living somewhere within my dramatic presentations. It was a thrilling possibility. There are times when one special audience member can add an element of total surprise. It's rare, but when it happens, the impact upon me as an actress, as well as upon the rest of the audience, can change the dynamic of my performance.

My presentation that evening, called "A Patriot's Heart," included five characters representing the American spirit. My third vignette was a portrayal of Mary Todd Lincoln. This woman's poignant and misunderstood life story is filled with such majesty and tragedy. Mary was a coquettish woman deeply in love with Mr. Lincoln, and I portray her as such. During my performance, I tell many of the charming stories that she would have told. They are rich stories, ones that open a window onto the courtship and family life that Mary so enjoyed with her beloved husband. At the beginning of this particular vignette, my goal is always to make the audience feel comfortable, safe, and warm—as they would feel if they were in their own homes.

But then, out of nowhere—wracking grief!

"Why! Why would they kill my husband?" she wails. "Why do they hate him so? I can't understand it. How can there be a world filled with so much hatred—such terrible hatred!"

Then suddenly, she splits the air with a shrill scream!

Yes, I have the audience in the palm of my hands. There's a collective gasp as they slide forward to the edge of their seats.

Mary Lincoln continues to cry out in despair. Her hands tremble uncontrollably as her body is bent into a tortuous position. She is on the verge of collapse.

What happens next I could not have scripted. As if on cue, my gallant gentleman in the first row stands and steps forward—one deliberate step after another. Now, facing a shocked audience, we are standing together. He extends his hand and looks at me with warm eyes. His face is filled with such deep sympathy and compassion.

As a professional actress, I have enjoyed, and on some occasions endured, numerous interruptions and unusual occurrences while performing. The stage can be a place of unexpected mystery for the actor as well as the audience. Invariably, these alterations build layers of experience for staying in character under all circumstances. But in my entire career before this, I had never faced such a potent mix of feelings: wonder, disquiet, fascination—and yet, no real concern.

Gently placing his left hand on my shoulder, my new compatriot softly said, "There, there. Everything's going to be all right." The audience was wide-eyed and frozen in place. Quickly gathering my thoughts and continuing in character, I reached over, took his hand in mine, and closed the distance between us.

We must have been a touching tableau: a small, slender white woman receiving solace from a tall, elegant black man. In spite of the ravages of Alzheimer's, he had stepped into the moment and offered a loving gesture of pure compassion to a woman in need. We had breached time and space, drawing past and present into one never-to-be-forgotten moment.

~Mary Margaret Mann

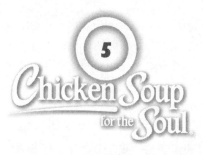

Me and the Night Don't Get Along

A mom's hug lasts long after she lets go.
~Author Unknown

My mom has Alzheimer's. It sucks. I think she is past the scariest part—realizing she is "losing her mind." When her symptoms first began to show, she was scared, paranoid, forgetful, and irritable. She knew something was happening. At first I thought it was just my mom being dramatic. But looking back a few years, her behavior was strange. And soon it became clear she was slipping away.

When she was in the early stage of the disease, I called to check in one evening and she said quietly, "Me and the night don't get along." My mother had never been afraid to go out alone at night. And she walked everywhere—she never had a driver's license. But now she needed someone with her all the time to feel safe.

"Me and the night don't get along"—that's quite the lyric. My mother was as witty as they come. She wrote tons of poems and parodies of songs. Mostly they were for co-workers leaving for another job, for castmates at the close of a show, or for my sisters' bosses or workmates. She would whip something up in an evening. She could do it all. Of course she had raised nine kids, too, which sums it up.

Now she's past the fear, and she's peaceful. She eats well and is in a nice nursing home. But it's still a nursing home. I think she still knows she has some kind of disease, but she has moments of peace.

I don't like to say *was* because she still *is*. She is still sweet and interested in what you're saying. Her quick wit is still there. The one-liners. Her laugh. Her wink. She can still sing all the "golden oldies" from the '40s and '50s verbatim.

And that's what makes me believe there is still a person in there. A light. A soul. A living, breathing, human being.

And that's what breaks my heart.

~Joey McIntyre

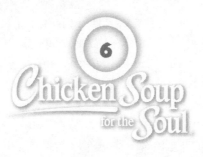

The Lady in the Mirror

The ultimate lesson all of us have to learn is unconditional love,
which includes not only others but ourselves as well.
~Elisabeth Kübler-Ross

One day I met the Lady in the Mirror. It began several years ago, after Mom had been diagnosed with Alzheimer's and was in an assisted living facility. I was helping her find some pants that fit, and she was trying them on and looking in the mirror. At the same time, we were talking about the people who worked in the facility and her friends there. I was having a hard time figuring out what was real and what wasn't in her side of the conversation.

She turned and said, "Well, her? I like her. She is always really nice to me."

Who was she talking about? "Her," she said, pointing to her reflection in the mirror.

It caught me so off guard. There we were doing normal things, and suddenly she was talking about her reflection as if it were another person. How should I react? I looked closely, as if there was going to be someone else in that mirror, and said, "Who, Mom?"

She again pointed at herself in the mirror and said, "Her. That nice lady."

"Great. I am so glad she's nice to you."

I learned long ago there is no arguing with someone with Alzheimer's. There is no bringing them back to reality. Once a piece of information is gone, it's gone. There is no relearning it as a child might. So I went along, still in a state of shock. It wasn't until later that I could accept that the lady in the mirror was real to Mom. I could see that for now, at least, the lady in the mirror was her normal, her truth—so it would have to be mine, too.

A few weeks later I went to visit Mom, and I found her in someone else's room trying to get some peace and quiet. Even my mom sometimes needs a break from the constant ruckus in the Alzheimer's ward—people yelling things that don't make sense, ladies trying to sell you their walkers and talking to dolls, one man giving lectures as he did when he was a professor.

That day she seemed tired and out of it. I asked if she wanted to walk around. She agreed, but soon she had to use the bathroom. When I went in to make sure she washed her hands, she was talking to someone in the mirror and I stopped to listen.

She asked, "Where is your brother?" and replied, "Isn't that nice, really?" to a voice only she could hear.

I interrupted to ask, "Mom, do you want to walk with me or would you rather stay here and talk?"

She replied, "Yeah, I am kinda busy right now. I think I'll stay here and talk." And so I was passed up for the lady in the mirror.

Another time I walked in to find Mom napping. I was going to leave her laundry and come back the next day, but just then, Mom woke up. "Hi Mom, it's me, Molly, your daughter." Since Mom may or may not recognize me when we meet, I always identify myself to her.

That day she remembered me and said, "Hi, hon. Come here, I want you to meet someone before they leave." And so I was reintroduced to the lady in the mirror. To my mother's reflection, no matter that mine was also peering back at us. I greeted her and that was enough for Mom.

No matter how many times things like this happen, they feel so utterly strange to me. My mom's reality, which constantly shifts to non-reality and back again, can be so confusing, even though I experience it constantly. One minute we can be talking to her reflection and introducing ourselves, the next she will touch my arm, as she always used to, and ask, "How are you and your husband doing?"

I am glad she loves her reflection, because she sees herself as a kind being. This is yet another lesson my mother has taught me out of the confusion that now is her life. We all should love the man or woman, boy or girl we see in the mirror. We should love ourselves with the kind of love my mom has for her lady in the mirror, even though she doesn't know she is seeing herself, my beautiful, loving, and kind Mom.

Look and see, and be as kind to yourself as the Lady in the Mirror is to my mother.

~Molly Godby

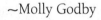

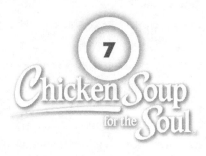

Black Eyebrows

It is a far, far better thing to have a firm anchor in nonsense
than to put out on the troubled seas of thought.
~John Kenneth Galbraith

"N o, you cannot have black. You're getting brown," I say to my eighty-six-year-old mother.

"But I want black!" she whines.

"Mom, you used to wear black when your hair was dark. It's white now, and brown is more suitable," I tell her as I walk with her to the cosmetics section. In my mind I see her face as it was a week ago, made up with stark black eyebrows haphazardly colored in by her hand.

Today she is using her cane and surprisingly able to keep up with me. A few weeks ago she would not have been able to. It's incredible what a shot of cortisone to the knee can do.

I pick up an eyebrow pencil in brown and show it to her. "How much is that one?" she asks.

"$5.99," I answer.

"Put it back. I don't want it," she says, walking to the next shelf.

I grab up another pencil and get the same question.

"$4.50," I tell her.

She waves a hand in the air. "No, I don't want that one either."

I find another brand for 99 cents. "Okay, I'll take that one," she says. "But don't they have the powder kind? That's what I really want."

I tell her no and direct her to the front of the store. My husband takes the shopping cart from me. He goes through the checkout while I sit on a bench with my mother. It's standard procedure when we take her shopping.

As we wait, my mother says something that reminds me of my father.

"You sound just like Dad," I say to her. "Except he would have said, 'What the hell's the difference?'" I'm laughing as I add in the swear word.

She smiles. "January 4th," she says as she moves her cane off to the side.

"What?"

"January 4th, the day he died," she answers.

"No Mom, July… July 6th," I tell her.

She looks at me quizzically, her bare eyebrows drawing close. "July? I thought it was January."

"No, Mom. July 6th."

"Oh. Well he's in a better place than we are."

It's her customary line. One she has used many times during the past two years.

I sit there and people watch. An obese woman is coming towards us. She sits in a motorized shopping cart, trying to maneuver it back to its mooring.

Quickly I turn to my mother. "So what did you do today?" I ask.

Too late. She has already spotted the woman. "Honey, look at that woman! Look how fat she is!" she says.

"Shh, don't say that, Mom," I whisper.

"Why? She can't hear me," she says in her normal tone.

She had always taught me not to stare at people because they were different.

I change the subject and breathe a sigh of relief when I distract her.

"So, January 4th," she says again.

"No, Mom. July 6th," I tell her and the whole conversation begins again.

She shakes her head and taps her index finger to her forehead. "Nobody home," she says.

We drive back to her house and sit on the front porch. I go inside and call my sister.

"We took her to Kmart. I bought her an eyebrow pencil," I tell Joanna.

"No!" she yells into the phone. "Have you seen what she looks like when she gets hold of an eyebrow pencil? She makes herself look like a clown!"

I laugh and tell her yes, I have seen her. "I felt bad not getting it for her," I say as I check my mother's pillbox.

"Don't give it to her. She'll forget you bought it anyway," Joanna says.

I agree to keep it for now.

I finish my conversation and go back outside to join my mother and husband.

"What are those?" my mother asks pointing to red roses on a bush.

"Mom, what do they look like?" I ask.

"A rose?" she asks.

I nod.

"Yeah a rose, but is there any other name for it?" she asks.

"A rose is a rose by any other name," my husband quotes. He is not into Shakespeare and I can tell by the way he says it that he has answered my mother many times already.

"And what's that?" she asks pointing to a solar lantern in the front garden.

"What does it look like?" I ask again.

"A light?" she asks.

"Yes, Mom, it's a light."

"Oh, so I pay for it with my electricity," she says with disgust.

"No Mom, it's solar. I bought it for Dad a few years ago."

She is quiet for a minute and I watch the boys a few doors down playing basketball.

"January 4th," she says again, this time staring off into space.

"Yeah Mom, January 4th," I answer.

~Maria Montagna Bohlman

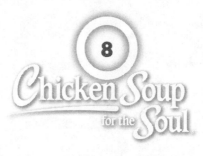

Slipping Away

Are you really sure that a floor can't also be a ceiling?
~M.C. Escher

Daily I watch as she gradually
slips away from me and all reality.
In her mind I have become young again.
She keeps admonishing me to come in
from the cold and have supper,
telling me that Daddy will soon
be home from work.
Daddy's been dead for ten years
but the reality of that has never
caught up with her.
I stifle tears, put on a smile, shout "I'm coming, Mom!"
and pretend to stamp my feet from the cold,
despite the summer heat.
Again I step into her world.

~Sue Young

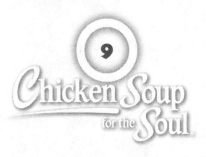

Good Times with Mom

If you want to be happy, be.
~Leo Tolstoy

My personal experience with Alzheimer's was my journey with my beloved mother, Eula Stanislaus. My mother was diagnosed with Alzheimer's disease in 2006. I had noticed some little changes in her prior to 2006, but because I didn't understand the early signs of the disease it went unnoticed.

I remember in 2003 Mom and I were walking in New York City, and we had just passed a bakery. Mom turned to me and said she didn't smell anything.

I looked at her and said, "Mom, you really can't smell that?"

"No, I really can't."

I accepted this and chalked it up to her getting older. She was seventy-two. Now I know that one of the signs of early-stage Alzheimer's might be as simple as not being able to smell peanut butter.

Then her hands began shaking uncontrollably and sometimes she could not get her legs to move when she wanted to get up and walk. It was as if she would send a signal from her brain to her legs but her legs wouldn't receive it. If only I had had more awareness and education about the disease, I could have helped her manage the symptoms in these very early stages.

As a caregiver, meeting the challenges of this everyday fight, with what I now realize was Alzheimer's, was devastating. I had not been aware of the challenges I would be up against and the continual devolution in my mother's ability to do anything for herself.

Mom sometimes didn't want to take her medicine; she didn't express hungriness; she was in a constant state of forgetfulness, and sometimes she would imagine little babies sitting in her living room, or she would call out for people who had been dead for more than forty years. I learned with this disease to expect the unexpected, to be prepared to go with the flow and to react calmly to whatever she was going through in that particular moment.

This was obviously a great deal for me to handle. It was emotional to watch my mom — my best friend — changing from an adult to someone more childlike. To watch her change into someone who I had to console through my tears by saying, "As long as I am caring for you, everything will be all right."

My mother's symptoms were such that I could still take her everywhere I went. I never left her behind. But for me, managing stress became harder as the disease progressed. My mom needed me more and more every day and the result was that I looked after myself less and less. I made this choice because I felt no one would or could take care of my mother as well as I could. It was the best choice I ever made, and without hesitation, I would make that same choice again.

On the brighter side, there were so many funny moments. My husband, two daughters, and I understood how to handle certain situations that cropped up again and again. If Mom saw those small babies in the living room, we would say, "Okay Mom, point out where they are so we don't sit on them." Then we would all laugh, including Mom.

Sometimes we would leave the room and when we came back, she would look at us as if it was the first time she had seen us all day. We would give her a big hug and announce we were home and so happy to see her. Mom would give us the biggest smile. No matter how many times we had to repeat the process she remained happy, a big smile plastered on her face.

Overall, my mom had a peaceful and loving experience as she

fought this disease. As a family, we made it fun for her. I would dress her up in bright outfits and comb her beautiful hair, which was down to her waist. I would have her nails done. Her make-up would be impeccable and she loved to wear her red lipstick. She dressed sharp every day and it made her feel good about herself. We took her out to dinner to beautiful places, as she always appreciated beauty. I always said because she was such a beautiful spirit, every day was a beautiful day for her.

~Bern Nadette Stanis

People living with early-stage
Alzheimer's have stated that one
of the most important lessons
they learned early on in their
diagnosis is this:
They could not just wait for
others to help them—they had to
go out and help themselves to
the best of their ability.

"You are not alone"
alz.org/ihavealz

Living
with Alzheimer's
& Other Dementias

What Does It Feel Like?

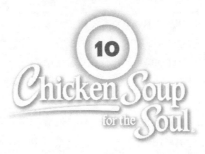

Remember Me

The purpose of life is a life of purpose.
~Attributed to both Ludwig Wittgenstein and Robert Byrne

I was a nurse for thirty years. Near the end of my career, I began to notice that I was struggling to complete daily tasks. There was always an excuse; I was tired or had worked too many hours. I began having trouble with my knee and took time off work to have surgery. It was during this time that I started to take note of my problems.

I had days that I called "lights on" or "lights off." When the lights were off I didn't know when or what I ate, I had no idea if I slept or how long I had slept. Verbal and written information was hard for me to understand, and I got lost in familiar places. If I only lost my keys on any given day that was a good day.

When the lights were "on" I had to clean the mess I had made while the lights were "off." Once, I went to wash clothes and there were no dirty clothes. I had been wearing dirty clothes for days, unaware of how long this had been going on.

In 2011, I found myself at a stop sign and I didn't know where I was or how I got there. In that moment I decided to make an appointment to see my doctor. I had an eight-year relationship with my primary care physician and felt she knew me really well. During my office visit, I cried while talking with the nurse, and my physician agreed that the changes I was experiencing were not like me.

My doctor referred me to a neurologist and on my sixty-third birthday, with my son at my side, I underwent testing and was diagnosed with Alzheimer's disease. My son asked questions, but I didn't. I was happy to know there was a word for my problem, and although I know how this disease will end, every day I wake up and accept who I am that day.

In May 2012, at the urging of my son and son-in-law, I moved into a residential community they both felt would be a good fit for me. I would be close to my family, my care team, and the specialists who conduct the clinical trial in which I am a participant. Yet, the most important part of my care team is my supportive children, and I was grateful to be closer to my son.

Shortly after moving, he spent Mother's Day with me and afterward he wrote me a letter. I cherish this part:

Mom, I don't want you to worry or be afraid. Let's enjoy every single day and not think too much about whether you can remember as well as you could in the past. I will watch over you and won't let anything bad happen to you. If the time comes when we need to do more for you, I will make sure you have everything you need to have a great quality of life. I wish I could change things. I wish I could take your illness for you and I can't. All I can do is be there for you and love you.

Yes, I have a loving and supportive family. I am a very positive person and if something starts to bother me I ask myself, "Does this really matter?"

I accept my disease and am proud to be a National Early-Stage Advisor for the Alzheimer's Association. I have made it my goal to inform the public that I live a great life with support from my family. I am very active, and I want to work to change the stigma associated with the word Alzheimer's. I have met so many wonderful professionals who have allowed me to share my story in an effort to educate others who are dealing with the effects of this disease. With the support of the Alzheimer's Association, I have advocated for the needs and rights of others with the disease.

I may be just one voice, but together with other advocates, we are unified.

To put an end to this fatal disease, we need to advocate for more research and clinical study participants. As a participant myself, I know I may not benefit from the studies, but someone else will—and thinking about that makes me smile.

As a legacy to my family, I want to be a part of a movement that educates others and helps advocate for people with Alzheimer's and their families. As this disease progresses, I won't remember anyone, but I want to live my life so that people will remember me.

~Cynthia A. Guzman

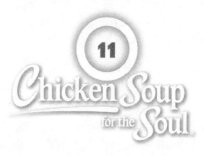

What My Alzheimer's Diagnosis Has Taught Me

With the past, I have nothing to do; nor with the future. I live now.
~Ralph Waldo Emerson

've always been the type of person who prefers experiences to things. I'd rather go on a trip and have great memories than buy a new computer. I enjoy time with my family, laughing at silly things, having coffee with a dear friend and taking a walk in my neighborhood. I like to do things that create memories.

How ironic then, that at age forty-six, I was diagnosed with Alzheimer's disease—a disease that robs you of your memories.

By being diagnosed at an early age, I was an anomaly to many. When people know you have Alzheimer's you become branded—it's like you have a big "A" stamped on your forehead. People treat you differently. They are not sure how to approach you. They don't know if you will remember them. They don't think you can speak for yourself. They don't think you have thoughts in your head.

Many times people come up to me and say, "You look great—you can't be sick." I wish that were true.

Seeing this reaction from people made me realize there were lots of misconceptions about Alzheimer's disease. Alzheimer's does not affect everyone the same way. There are different rates of progression, different symptoms, and different ways to manage symptoms. What works for one may not work for others.

I realized I had an opportunity to help educate people about this disease. I needed to show them that, for now, I am *living* with Alzheimer's disease, not *dying* from it. I am still a wife, a mother, a mother-in-law, sister, an aunt, and a friend. I need to be those things for as long as I can.

Many families don't want to admit that a loved one has Alzheimer's. That's certainly their right. I've never been ashamed of it. People don't seem to be ashamed of other diseases like diabetes or high blood pressure. I do, however, feel guilt—guilt for what this disease means for my family.

I have the easy part, they have the hard part—they have to live with me. My behavior is unpredictable. Many times I know I am not making sense to them but I can't fix it. I know I am not doing something right, but I can't stop myself. My thoughts get trapped in my brain with no way to get out. It's frustrating for me but much more so for my family.

The brain is a complex thing. It is hard to understand when your brain doesn't work. Some days my brain works fine. Some days it doesn't. I don't know when my brain is going to work and when it isn't.

We take it for granted that it is going to work the same way it always has and when it doesn't, frustration builds. I get agitated. I get mad. I feel alone. I feel stupid. I know I'm not stupid, but when you can't do a task you have done for years, you feel stupid. I always thought I was in control of my life, and now Alzheimer's is in control.

I've learned a lot since the day of my diagnosis—not only about the disease but also about myself. I've always known that life is what you make it, but I never lived it that way. Now I do.

To cope with this monster, my family and I decided that we would look at Alzheimer's as an obstacle in our life, rather than the end of my life. We decided that when I could no longer do something, we would look for another way to do it for as long as possible. I've learned to live in the moment.

It saddens me that there are many tomorrows I will never know and many yesterdays I cannot remember. So today is what I have. I used to worry about what was, or how I should have done something differently. But that is energy wasted. I need all of my energy to get through every day.

I've learned to slow down and pace myself. I've learned to rest when I need to—it gives my brain a chance to recharge. I've learned that routine is important and I do best in a quiet environment. I've learned to plan my days better. I need to live my life as normally as possible, knowing that the definition of normal often changes. Some days are perfect. Other days are a disaster. Some days I laugh at the crazy things I do. Other days I cry at the crazy things I do.

I've learned to rely on others. It isn't easy asking for help, but sometimes I have to. Admitting that I can no longer do something and having to ask someone for help is humbling. I've learned to let go of the things I can no longer do and hold tightly to those I still can. There will be a day when I will hardly be able to do anything, and I hope for my sake and the sake of my family that it is well into the future.

I've learned to share my journey. If others can learn from my experiences, all the better. I'll talk to whoever will listen and I chronicle my adventures in a blog: www.creatingmemories.blogspot.com.

I've learned to stay active—physically and mentally. I spend countless hours working on puzzles and trying my hand at crafting—anything to keep the brain going. I also try to eat right and exercise on a regular basis. I notice a dip in my mental acuity when I don't exercise.

I've learned to laugh at myself and to ask others to laugh with me. Laughing also helps eliminate those awkward moments when people don't know how to react to something you've done.

I've learned to prioritize. My family and friends are first. Everything else is last. I know I can't stop Alzheimer's, but maybe I can help change its direction.

I've learned to keep adding to my bucket list. My lifelong dream of going to Australia with my family was fulfilled. In time, I know I will forget that trip, but I hope my family will remember it forever.

In the future, I hope research will find a way to conquer this dreaded disease. I hope you will never have to take this same journey, but if you do, try to make the best of this bad situation and try to enjoy what is left of a "normal" life for as long as you can.

~Kris Bakowski

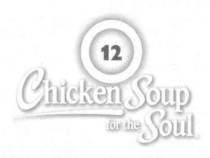

Coping with Alzheimer's

I believe the future is only the past again, entered through another gate.

~Arthur Wing Pinero

Many years ago, I worked as a psychologist for the Navy's Military Sealift Command. Toward the end of my last tour of duty, I visited Ryoanji, the famous Buddhist monastery and meditation rock garden in Kyoto, Japan. Although I found the rock garden cultivated a sense of calm stillness within me, I gained the greatest spiritual insight as I left.

Along the path there was a small sign reading "The Usual Path." It was meant to direct tourists back to their destination. The sign did not read, "The Right Path" or "The Only Path," just "The Usual Path."

Most tourists opted for the usual path. It was safe and predictable, while the unusual path was unfamiliar and filled with challenges. But ultimately both paths led to the same place. That small, unbiased sign in the Buddhist monastery garden has given me inspiration and courage on my alternative path as a person living with Alzheimer's.

When first diagnosed with younger-onset Alzheimer's disease, it became crystal clear to me that I was no longer on "The Usual Path." My journey now is unusual, unfamiliar, and full of challenges — both for me and my loved ones. When first diagnosed, my life as I knew it, and the plans I had for it, changed. I have no idea how long my memory and cognitive functions will serve me.

My experience coping with Alzheimer's is similar to others who have been diagnosed with this disease. Suddenly, I had to navigate life insurance policies, trusts, wills, financial and long-term care planning, early retirement, social security disability, state disability insurance, medical directives, and compromised health—all at the same time. This journey has been nothing short of overwhelming and confounding.

The longer I am on this journey, the more I have a sense of urgency to live life to the fullest. I am "seizing the moment." Ironically, I am happier now than I ever have been, mindful of the present moment rather than worrying about the future or brooding about the past. Prior to my Alzheimer's diagnosis, much of my life was about striving for this or that and not really paying attention to the things I value most—my primary and secondary relationships, spirituality, and health.

Being mindful of the present moment is a beneficial way to deal with the daily health and emotional challenges of this disease. The capability to live in the present moment deepens, develops, and matures when there is an intention to pay attention. Daily walking (or some sort of exercise) also helps, because it is a deliberate exercise to strengthen body, mind, and spirit.

My choice is to be a fighter and not a victim of Alzheimer's. To have the energy to fight a good fight, I need to renew, rekindle, and rediscover my inner spirit. And the only way I know to do this is by seizing the moment, cultivating stillness and quiet, avoiding stimuli and distractions, and embracing the value and meaning of life. Because of Alzheimer's, not in spite of it.

~Lou A. Bordisso, Ed.D.

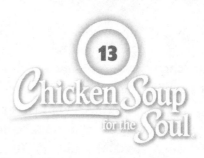

Socializing Amidst Mental Chaos

I am not afraid of storms for I am learning how to sail my ship.
~Louisa May Alcott

t was nearing midnight on August 25, 2012, exactly seventy-eight years and twenty-four hours since my birth at Grandmother's house in West Virginia. Six hours ago I had entered the banquet room at Galaxy Restaurant in Wadsworth, Ohio, and met a sea of aging faces, some familiar, others less so—classmates from Copley High School's class of 1952.

Tony, a man who has aged better than most of us, greeted me with a big smile and an anecdote I struggled to interpret. "Glad you could make it, Lois," he said. "I think of you every time I drive through the Shenandoah Valley in Virginia."

Greeting him, I smiled, trying to assimilate the meaning of his remark.

He explained to a bystander that a few years ago, as I had left the Shenandoah Valley, driving up the mountainside, my phone rang and a voice had announced bluntly to me that tests showed I had Alzheimer's disease. I had that story published in *Chicken Soup for the Soul: Think Positive*, and I also included it in my book about my first twelve months with my diagnosis, *Essays: On Living with Alzheimer's Disease, The First Twelve Months*. So now I get it. He read my story.

Others who had read my book approached me, remarking about

how well I looked, and how they couldn't believe I have Alzheimer's because I look and sound so good. Tony thought perhaps I made up the entire story.

Reflecting on the scene, I found I agreed with them in many ways; yet I didn't feel very well this particular night. Still I'd ponied up and put on a happy face, determined to be at my best. I gained confidence after a shower, slipping into a new outfit and having my granddaughter do my hair—thinking that after sixty years, I could finally hold my own with anyone in this group.

These old feelings of inferiority stemmed from high school, when I joined the class after the school term started, coming from southern Appalachia without social skills or friends. I never quite overcame the lack of equality even after accomplishing more educationally and professionally than most of my class members. As the years passed, I realized they had accepted me all along; some even admired me in later years.

The restrictions were set in place by my own lack of confidence; it's strange that it wasn't until I had dementia that I made the association.

The self-confident feeling didn't last all evening. I cringed when I started to the restroom, turning the wrong direction. I returned and forgot which of three closed double doors opened into our banquet room. Embarrassed when I realized I opened the wrong door, I turned around and noted "Class of '52" printed on the doors I had just passed.

I was able to endure the first two hours of the social evening quite well. My strategy was to talk to the people who had been my friends in school, who I had contact with and reason to remember in more recent times. When subjects came up that I should have known about, I smiled and nodded as if I understood. In other instances, I asked questions, which revealed my lack of knowledge. My classmates either didn't notice, or pretended not to.

Regardless of my planning or how much I rest prior to an event, once I start getting tired—usually after two hours or so—the confusion and poor memory take over. Then I know it's time to get to the safety of home and family. On this evening, I started counting the minutes until my daughter would drive me home, where I could close my eyes and relax. I wanted to feel safe again.

What a pretender I am! I'm fortunate to be able to put on a good act — and the reunion was my best performance in a long time — but it just doesn't last.

How does one socialize when living with Alzheimer's disease? Very carefully, and with much anxiety!

~Lois Bennett

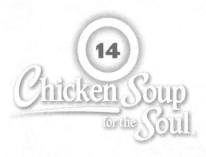

What Alzheimer's Disease Feels Like

I am only one, but I am one. I cannot do everything, but I can do something.
And I will not let what I cannot do interfere with what I can do.
~Edward Everett Hale

t was an uncharacteristically warm and sunny morning in Alaska. I was sitting on the aft deck of a cruise ship watching brilliant blue icebergs drift silently by, on vacation with my partner Candy. We had decided to go on a seven-day cruise through Alaska's Inside Passage because I had always wanted to see the glaciers and time was running out.

Diagnosed six years ago with Alzheimer's disease at age sixty, it was time for me to do those lifetime adventures. As I watched one small iceberg glisten in the sunlight, I was drawn to its facets and how as each one caught the sunlight a small piece would topple off. This is what it's like to have this disease, I thought. My brain is the iceberg and every day I lose some little part of it. There are days when the sun is bright and I may lose a bigger or more obvious piece and there are cloudy, cold days when I don't lose anything. Such is the life of an iceberg and a brain attacked by Alzheimer's disease.

When I was first diagnosed, it had become apparent to me that I was having cognitive problems. Once a creative, holistic thinker, I could no longer hold in my head the many ideas needed for this type of thinking. I had become much more linear in my approach to life.

Now Step 1 had to be followed by Step 2 and then 3. I could write these steps down and follow them at least most of the time. As my symptoms progress and I lose more and more, I have come to appreciate one aspect of this disease—forgetting. Every time I am aware of a change in my abilities it is only apparent for a short time. During that time I become distressed, but I know that in a very short time I won't remember ever having it. I guess this is a protective process, and it does make life easier for me.

Our vacation was different for me this time. I knew that what I was experiencing was spectacular but I missed its intensity. It's as if the colors of the sky or a sunset or the blues of the glacier were all grayer. There was still color and beauty, but it was just not the same.

As a psychologist, I learned that we store our memories in many different places in our brains. Often a smell or taste will elicit a powerful memory, even though the image has long been forgotten. Every night I'd try to recall what I'd seen that day. It was difficult. Realizing this, I tried to create mental postcards and absorb the smells, tastes, and sounds of the places we went.

When I reflect on what I have lost, I am still aware of two important things. One is my intelligence and creative drive; the other is my connection to others. Both of these have changed dramatically and I miss them greatly. Always a self-motivated (and some would say driven) person, I now need other people to help me find ways to be helpful to others. I have gone from being the person others went to for ideas and direction to being directed. This has changed my relationships in major ways.

I have had to learn to depend on my family and colleagues, which has taught me the value of joining. Although my bond with other people has diminished, I still want to be useful and productive—I just don't always know how anymore. This disease has humbled me. It has given me a new understanding of myself and the world of others. I believe that with any chronic progressive illness, we are presented with moments of insight and opportunity. What we do with them defines us in ways we might never have imagined.

I have chosen empowerment over victimization, which I believe has contributed to my slow rate of decline.

The German philosopher Martin Heidegger wrote, "Anyone can achieve their fullest potential.... who we are might be predetermined, but the path we follow is always of our own choosing. We should never allow our fears or the expectations of others to set the frontiers of our destiny. Your destiny can't be changed but it can be challenged. Every man is born as many men and dies as a single one."

I intend to be the author of this chapter of my life and actively shape the man I will die as.

~Dr. Stephen Hume

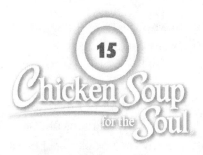

Living Well with Alzheimer's

The important thing is not how many years in your life
but how much life in your years.
~Edward J. Stieglitz

My name is Carmen Cruz and I am seventy-seven years old. Two years ago, I was diagnosed with early-stage Alzheimer's disease. A few years prior, I noticed that I was forgetting parts of my daily routine, and was tested. To my relief, the results were negative. A year later, I again noticed bouts of forgetfulness, only this time they were more frequent. Again I requested the appropriate tests, and this time, it was confirmed that I had early signs of Alzheimer's disease.

In my younger years, this disease was virtually unknown—or it at least didn't carry the same name. In the small pueblos of Puerto Rico where I grew up, persons with these symptoms were called crazy and were institutionalized. Thankfully, times have changed.

Now that I've read vast amounts of material on the disease and its progression, my opinion is that the disease itself is a criminal. In a competition with the most unlawful and immoral villain, Alzheimer's would win because it is a careful, heartless thief. Its only aim is to steal from its victims—their memories, rationality, and thoughts.

Despite Alzheimer's intention to rob me of my experiences, I have triumphed since my diagnosis. I didn't take the time to sit, lament, and wait for each stage of the disease to take its toll.

The first thing I did was to accept my reality. I ingested all the information I could find, listened to the doctor's recommendations, and committed to living them out. I am determined to fight, the opposite of what the disease wants me to do. And with my family's support, I continue each day living life to the fullest of my abilities.

I've bought many books and crosswords, things to stimulate my brain, and I spend hours on end diving into these tasks. Upon being diagnosed, I made it my goal to write the story of my life and I managed to complete this task in one year's time, accounting for my life from six years old until today. It was an incredible effort; I put my mind to work in overdrive.

Today, I am invested in scrapbooking with hundreds of pictures I have saved over the years. So far, I have made two for my daughter, two for my son, and I am in the process of completing one for myself. My goal is to start my three grandchildren's scrapbooks when mine is complete, if my mind permits. This is the lifestyle that has helped me deal with Alzheimer's. I'm fortunate that in my situation, the disease is progressing extremely slowly.

The final stage may be unavoidable, and as human beings, we can only do so much. However, an Alzheimer's diagnosis is not the time to grieve and miss out on the remaining years of life. In consciously pursuing enjoyable tasks that put your mind to work, you make the most of the life you have, adding faith, exercises, and hope to the mix.

~Carmen Cruz

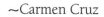

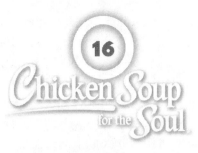

16

It's a Wonderful Life and Alzheimer's

The best part of life is not just surviving, but thriving with passion and compassion and humor and style and generosity and kindness.
~Maya Angelou

My favorite movie has always been *It's a Wonderful Life*. I love that George Bailey gets to see the impact he's had on so many people.

I was around ten or twelve years old when I first saw the movie. The story has always been a reminder that doing something good for others because you care—and not expecting anything in return—is one of life's greatest rewards.

This past July, at fifty-two years old, I was diagnosed with younger-onset Alzheimer's. It occurred to me that one of the things Alzheimer's does to a person is rob him of his memories, which is sort of what George Bailey went through. He got to see firsthand how no one recognized him: They knew nothing of his life, he had no friends, and, worse, he had no family.

That's kind of what is going to happen to me—only of course I will be the one not remembering anything. I know there are people who have a much worse lot in life. I only write this so that someone may relate to my perception of the disease.

Imagine never having been born; think of having all your memories taken away from you. I would not wish that on anyone. I still want to be the person I was before I received the diagnosis—a George Bailey kind of person. So I've decided to be an advocate for dementia awareness, specifically younger-onset Alzheimer's. I'm hoping to help get the word out that this disease doesn't only affect the elderly, as many people think. There are more than 200,000 people in the United States younger than age sixty-five affected by this disease.

I know I am the luckiest guy in the world. I found my one true love early in life, and we've been married for thirty-two years. We have an incredible family: two beautiful from-the-inside-out daughters who are married to two wonderful men, and a strong, caring, determined sixteen-year-old son who couldn't make a man more proud. And we have three gorgeous grandchildren.

So, just like George Bailey, I know I've had a wonderful life and will continue to make as many wonderful memories as I can. And I will try to remember, as Clarence said in the movie, "No man is a failure who has friends."

~Michael R. Belleville

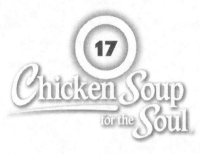

17

He Led the Way

Reason is our soul's left hand, Faith her right.
~John Donne

I couldn't focus. I couldn't remember people's names. I couldn't figure out how to do things that I had done every day forever. I've been a nurse for more than thirty-five years, but it felt like I could no longer do my job. I thought I must be stressed or tired or maybe burned out. After meeting with my boss, I had no choice but to admit what she had already witnessed. Something was wrong and I needed to find out what it was.

After a multitude of tests and several brain scans, I sat in my doctor's office awaiting the results. "I just need some time off," I assured myself. "Then I will get back to normal." But it wasn't to be.

At age fifty-five, my doctor informed me that I had younger-onset Alzheimer's disease. I can't remember much else he said that day. I walked out of his office with a prescription in hand and a book called *Surviving Alzheimer's*.

When telling my grandsons, Sawyer, ten, and Hudson, seven, I tried to say it in a way they could understand. Hudson assured me, "Don't be afraid, Gramma. I know you forget sometimes, but I think your memories are in a box in your brain and we just have to find the right key to open the box."

I had always enjoyed walking the boys to school, but as my illness progressed, I found that sometimes I would get turned around and find myself lost. It was difficult for me to ask for help, so instead I explained to the boys that I couldn't walk with them anymore.

"Wait, I have a solution," Hudson said. Yes, he used the word "solution"! The next day as we walked to school, every time we turned a corner he would make an arrow with a magic marker on the sidewalk showing me the way home. Sometimes I would cry just from the joy of these little boys.

After my diagnosis, each Thursday my sister Colleen and I attended an Alzheimer's Association support group. I would meet in one room with others who had the disease while she would talk with other caregivers.

As I was sitting with my group I started to feel cold. I could see our car, where my nice warm sweater was, from the window. So instead of asking for help, I thought I could quickly run down to the car, get my sweater and come right back.

Obviously I wasn't thinking clearly because when I got to the car of course it was locked. Then when I turned around to head back every building looked exactly the same. I didn't want to panic. I tried to stay calm. But I got confused and couldn't even remember if I had crossed the street.

I started to walk from building to building, hoping to find a sign that would help lead me back to the Alzheimer's Association. Unfortunately there was none. Which way to turn, I didn't know. What I did know was that I was cold and lost.

If I were to describe how it feels for me to be lost, I would say that my body and mind are wrestling for control. My body thinks it knows where to go, so my instinct is to keep walking. But my mind knows better. It wants to think and make a plan. For me that part is blank. I feel it in there but I can't seem to coax the information out. It's like having your memory, your decision-making skills, and the ability to go the right way always on the tip of your tongue.

I wasn't thinking anymore, so I kept walking. It was getting colder and I had no idea how long I had been gone. It seemed like it was a long time and I was certain my sister was worried sick.

I started to think about God and how He has been by my side

giving me strength to get through so many obstacles. As I continued to walk, it finally dawned on me to ask Him for help guiding me to safety.

As I kept walking I saw a building up ahead. Once I got close enough I could see that I was looking at the back of the building, and when I looked up I noticed a small white object on the roof. I couldn't make out what it was but it seemed to be glowing. By now I was so confused I didn't trust my mind or my sight. But sure enough, as the building drew near, I saw a small white star glowing on the top of the roof.

If I hadn't been looking up, I might have missed it. A sense of calm came over me as I walked toward the star. I still didn't know what the building was but I continued on.

As I turned the corner I realized it was a church. I found a door and quickly opened it. The warmth hit me first, making me realize how cold I was after my long walk. A woman with a kind smile stood from behind her desk and asked, "Can I help you?"

I was crying. I couldn't speak. Not sure of my words or my name. The only words I managed to get out were, "I saw your star." She got a quizzical look on her face and said, "Just a moment." Another woman came in and she introduced herself as Reverend Snowden.

A few more jumbled words came out in between my tears and they finally figured out where I had come from and quickly called the Alzheimer's Association. After an emotional reunion with my sister, I went to thank Reverend Snowden.

She said, "Although it is very frightening to lose your way, it always feels better knowing that the road back is easier if you ask for help."

"I finally realized I had to ask for help," I said. "Once I accepted that, God was there to help me. And miraculously the star on your roof led me right to your door!"

"What star?" the reverend asked.

~Ann Marie Skerl

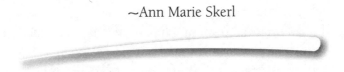

A person with dementia will
eventually need assistance with
daily living. By using creativity
and caregiving skills, you can
adapt routines and activities as
needs change.

"Daily Care"

alz.org/care

Chapter 3

Living with Alzheimer's & Other Dementias

Strategies and Tips for Coping

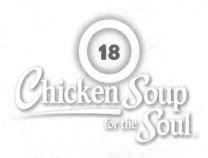

The ABC's of Alzheimer's and Dementia for Caregivers

Approach with a positive attitude, from the front, with a smile. Address the person with the disease by name.

Breathe. Take a deep breath before the visit/encounter. The person will read your essence and body language before he or she can comprehend what you are saying.

Cue the person. Instead of asking "Do you want to put on your sweater?" put yours on and offer to help.

Dementia is a general term for a decline in mental ability severe enough to interfere with daily life. Alzheimer's is the most common type of dementia, diagnosed 60-80 percent of the time.

Every day is a new day. A bad day yesterday does not mean a bad day today. Take it one day at a time.

Follow the lead. If the person with dementia wants to tell the same story or wash the same dish over and over again, let them.

Give the person a purpose. Ask for advice or give him/her a task. Even if it is done wrong, the person will feel worthy and useful.

Honor who the person is now—and who he or she was before the disease.

Investigate. If the person is agitated, he or she may not be able to tell you why. Is she hungry or thirsty? Tired? Does he have to go to the bathroom?

Joy. Revel in the joyful moments. Let those moments fill you up.

Keep eye contact. It establishes trust and helps you make a connection.

Love. Give a lot of love. It makes the person feel safe and cared for.

Mistakes. You will make them. You will say and do the wrong things. Forgive yourself—caregiving is a very hard job.

Never argue with the person with dementia. It causes agitation for both of you and makes everything harder.

Oxygen. Like on an airplane, take your oxygen first. Care for yourself. If you are not a strong, healthy caregiver, you cannot be strong for the person with the disease.

Practice patience. It can take someone with dementia longer to understand your question and come up with an answer.

Quiet. TV, radio, and several conversations at once make it hard for the person to concentrate. Go to a quiet place to visit or connect.

Redirect. If the person is frustrated or upset, try changing the topic or environment. Suggest a favorite activity, or offer some tea or ice cream.

Simple. Keep sentences simple to facilitate communication.

Talk about things from the past. Recent memories will fade more quickly.

Use fiblets. "I have to pick up my daughter from school!" says the eighty-year-old. "Your daughter called, she is staying late to play soccer. Let's go in here and listen to some music..." Tell a little "fib" and then redirect the conversation.

Validate feelings and thoughts. "Yes, it is Tuesday (even if it's Friday) but today we are going to do a Friday activity." Do not tell the person that he or she is wrong.

Walk in the person's shoes. He or she is frustrated by this disease, too.

e**X**ercise. Go for a walk with the person or do chair exercises. Staying active is good for everyone.

You are not alone. The Alzheimer's Association has many resources to help, including a 24/7 Helpline (800-272-3900), support groups and caregiving courses. Reach out.

Zzzz's. Let the person rest. This disease is exhausting. For both of you. You rest too.

~Kristen Cusato
former Southwest Regional Director,
Alzheimer's Association Connecticut Chapter

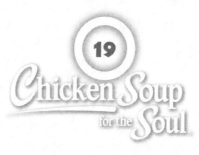

How I Learned to Lie

A little inaccuracy sometimes saves tons of explanation.
~Saki

And in the beginning, there I was… a fairly nice person with an excellent sense of ethics; kind to others, both human and four-legged; brought up properly; good manners; church-going; good values; helpful; polite; and always, always honest.

Then I learned to lie — and it felt good!

My mother's journey through her dementia altered my preconceived, well-established viewpoints on many things. As her dementia progressed, she began to travel first class down the road marked "Delusions," with dynamic side trips to the land of "Obstinate Refusal."

How was I to know in advance what this was going to mean to my belief system? Flying by the seat of my pants was my new mode of travel; there were many stopovers and the tickets were nonrefundable.

Delusions are rigid false beliefs and Mom had them in glorious abundance — this was her reality. She was amazingly good at embroidering around the edges of the imaginary fabric she wove and I had to enter her world, as she certainly was not able to function in mine.

She became delusion driven, filled with turmoil in her false beliefs. I stole all of her money. I was hiding the mail. I hid or stole her stamps. All I bought was rotten food. I hid her favorite bedspread.

I used her money to fly to Europe and buy jewels. I threw away her favorite clothes and purposely bought only the worst toilet paper. And, she did not wet the incontinence undergarments, somebody poured water on them. Yes, indeed.

I tried to explain, to accommodate, mollify, plead, and grovel. I was especially good at groveling.

One exhausting day, my wits had completely left me and Mom once again railed at me about my taking her good toilet paper and substituting "the cheap junk." Instead of explaining, pointing out, trying to educate or argue, I wistfully said in a weak voice, "I'll do better next time and buy the good stuff."

Expecting a thermonuclear explosion, I girded myself for the blast and fallout. But something strange happened. She stopped ranting, became calm and moved on. Huh? What?

Okay—let's try that again. A few days later, there was another delusional accusation fueled with agitation, "Gosh Mom, it must feel terrible when that happens, I will watch out for that." And again, there it was, the same outcome with return to calmness. I was on to something!

This is when my lying began in earnest and it was awesome in its rewards. The fixation on rotten food was from time to time a hugely difficult problem because then Mom would not eat. But by now, I was such a good liar, there ought to have been a medal.

"Let me get rid of that and go to the grocery store and get some fresh food." So, there I stood, putting various items from the refrigerator into plastic grocery bags and pretending I was taking them out to the garbage. I waited outside for ten minutes or so and re-entered the house with the same bags and same items, happily declaring, "Hi Mom, I got some really wonderful stuff at the market; so fresh and on sale, too!" I proceeded to put the same items back into the refrigerator and she was happy.

Initially, it was difficult for me to lie; I felt as though the earth might open up and swallow me for some of my whoppers. But as I developed insight, I came to understand that these fibs were a great kindness and not a moral lapse.

Later I learned this intervention is called "therapeutic fibbing." It was one of the best tools in my caregiving toolbox. These fiblets kept Mom from becoming agitated or having unnecessary meltdowns, which made her life so much better.

When Mom demanded we go somewhere, but there was no time, or it was stormy, or the middle of the night, I would say the car battery was dead and I had to wait until tomorrow for the garage man to come.

She insisted on controlling the remote control for her heating system and would crank it up to stifling. There was a spare controller so I took that one for myself and took the batteries out of hers. I told her that she was "now in charge of the heating system." She loved clicking that darned thing and it gave her great satisfaction. There was so much out of her control in her compromised life that this small bit of ersatz control was a delight for her.

If she refused a doctor's appointment, I would pretend it was for me and she just came along, or that the doctor could not refill her treasured blood pressure pills until he saw her and, by the way, we would stop for ice cream on the way home.

Was this always perfect? No, not always, but it was for the vast majority of the time. It kept my mother from having to suffer the irritability, agitation, and upset from the false beliefs her compromised brain was inducing. It was so, so much better.

As I grew in knowledge, I learned that my lies were actually "validating her feelings," and not her words. That made sense, as she was driven by her feelings. I also learned that when I validated what she was feeling it brought her comfort because she was being heard. And when I swiftly changed the subject after validating her feelings, that was called "re-focusing," and permitted me to move her from the delusion onto something more pleasant and comforting.

Therapeutic fibbing worked so well through our journey that I now recommend it to friends who have a loved one with dementia. Who knew lying could be ethical? One more lesson in life that not all things are written in stone. It was worth all of the prevarication to see Mom calm and even smiling. It all goes into the basket called quality of life.

~Johanna Richardson

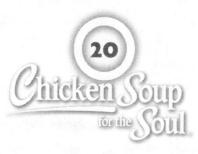

The Clock with One Hand

Our wedding was many years ago. The celebration continues to this day.
~Gene Perret

fell in love with the lady more than fifty years ago. We were both in high school. She's the gal I took to the prom. We dated through high school, we went off to different colleges but dated when we were back home for summers and holidays, and we got married right after college graduation.

We certainly had a happy, fulfilling, wonderful life together. We lived in Europe for a few years. We both got advanced degrees when we returned to the States. She taught English at the university and I had a rewarding business career. We raised two wonderful sons who now have families and careers of their own.

Throughout our lives there was always a division of duties. Nothing formal. We never really talked much about it; it just evolved. She took care of certain things and I took care of others. We handled just about everything as a close-knit team.

About eight years ago our world started to change. She noticed it before anyone else. She started to lose vocabulary. Occasionally she would have trouble explaining a concept to a student. Eventually it got to the point where she felt she couldn't teach at the level that her students deserved, and she gave up her teaching position.

My life started to change at that point, too. I tried to help her find the words she had lost. "That path along the side of the road is called a sidewalk." "The thing letters go in is called a mailbox." Dealing with a menu in a restaurant was difficult. She was losing the ability to read words, but even when I'd read the menu to her she didn't know fish from chicken. Once the entrée had been decided, I helped her choose sides with a piece of paper I kept in my wallet that had photos of baked, French fried, and mashed potatoes.

It was hard, but it was something I was happy to do for the love of my life. As her dementia worsened, our division of duties underwent drastic changes, and has now reached the point where if something has to be done, I do it. The marriage vows we made to each other those many years ago included "love, honor, and support," "in sickness and in health," and "till death do us part."

I'm glad I had a chance to share those vows with my wife. I count myself lucky to have shared all those years with her. Little did I know what those vows might involve, but I can say with all honesty that had I known I still would have made the vow, and knowing what I know today, I'm very glad that I did. At some point I will need to enlist even more help with my wife's day-to-day care. But until that day comes, I keep reminding myself that helping her dress, helping her eat, or carrying photographs of potatoes to help her decide side orders are all ways I can tell her that she is still the love of my life.

Since numbers have no meaning any longer, both digital and analog clocks are simply a source of puzzlement to her. Yet I often wish I could communicate to her the passage of time. How does one tell someone who has lost language that lunchtime isn't for an hour and a half, or that bedtime is in two hours?

I've developed a solution that seems to work. I bought a battery-powered wall clock and removed the second hand and the minute hand. She has become aware that although the remaining hour hand appears stationary, it does in fact move with time. Now I can put a piece of tape at the location the hand will be when it is dinnertime or bedtime, and she can check it occasionally to see that the hour hand is approaching the designated time.

Life certainly is full of twists and turns. Who would have thought that building a one-handed clock could be yet another way to tell my wife "I love you."

~Fred Kinsinger

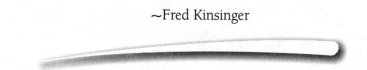

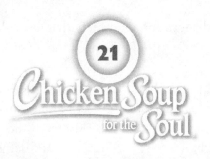

Mom and Her Foot Soldiers

We cannot live only for ourselves.
A thousand fibers connect us with our fellow men.
~Herman Melville

For my mom, life had become a never-ending war. She fought with my dad to take a weekly shower, they stayed hunkered-down in their house most of the time like they were stuck in a foxhole, and sometimes she had to map out her battle plan like a general in charge of troops.

"Sweetie, it's time to go to bed. Now!"

"Ollie, you spilled some soup on your shirt. Let's go and change it."

"Dearheart, you missed a pill. Take it now, please."

Unfortunately, my parents lived in Florida and I was stuck in the Midwest, too far away to help. Almost on the brink of collapsing, my mom was desperate.

We talked several times a week on the phone. I tried to fill my mother's life—for the duration of each long-distance conversation—with the small, light details of our lives. Her granddaughter's winning slide into home plate. Her grandson's most recent trumpet lesson. The antics of my third-grade students. For those few moments, she could forget her problems as she chuckled and cheered.

The disease that was draining my father's brain was incurable. Physically, however, he was teetering on the undefeatable. With every exam came the doctor's announcement that he could live another ten or twenty years. Unless things changed my mom would not last that long.

Together, she and I brainstormed some possible ways for her to get some respite. The idea of a nursing home was dismissed, as my dad still had some lucid moments. My mom did not want to miss the occasional glimmers of the husband and father he used to be. We considered hiring a part-time caregiver. Luckily, an Alzheimer's support group offered some wonderful solutions.

During the first few meetings Mom attended, a neighbor came over and stayed with my dad. Then the leader of the group told her about a day program. Once a week—on the day the support group met—members of a church cared for those with Alzheimer's. The families got a brief break while those with the disease received lunch and a snack, engaged in singing lessons, and painted with a local art teacher. There was a nominal fee, but the rewards were priceless.

Gentle and patient, the folks at the day care program didn't get frazzled when my dad dug in his heels. After they got to know him, they seemed to find my father's little temper tantrums amusing. He'd go off on a tangent, and they'd joke with him as they put an arm around him and nudged him down the hall to where he needed to go.

During a summer visit, I got to tag along and sit beside my mom during her meeting. She bubbled over about how much it was helping her, so I wanted to see for myself what was going on. Surrounding a table was a collection of wives and husbands and even a sibling, all worn out, but all obviously grateful to be able to vent about issues they all understood.

Listening to their stories, I was struck by how strong these people were. This was supposed to be a time when they could sit in side-by-side rocking chairs and hold hands as husband and wife. It was meant to be a time when they could laugh over the decades of memories they shared. But now, instead of partners who supported and assisted each other, one had become the caregiver—and their shifts never ended.

During the years that my mother went to those support group meetings, she was guided along the path by those who had navigated it before her. Mom learned the ins and outs of insurance and nursing homes. She picked up on some routines that would make my dad more comfortable as he became less and less coherent. Most importantly, though, for a couple of hours every week, my mother could sit down, relax, and share with others who had the same struggles.

This she did for herself. She realized it was crucial she give herself permission to take time for herself. After Mom joined the support group, she said on more than one occasion, "If I don't take care of myself, and I collapse, I can't take care of your dad."

While my mother uplifted and cared for Dad, her support group became her pillar, her army, preventing her from becoming a casualty in the war she waged against Alzheimer's.

~Sioux Roslawski

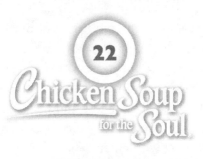

Living Without Math

Mathematics are well and good but
nature keeps dragging us around by the nose.
~Albert Einstein

recently took a good, hard look at myself in the mirror. My eyelids are beginning to sag over my blue eyes. My ruddy sun-damaged skin is going slack around my ears. I have a lone freckle on my plump bottom lip.

"Hi Dad," I said to my forty-seven-year-old reflection. "I'd recognize you anywhere."

Long before my father died of complications associated with Alzheimer's disease, people frequently remarked on our similar appearance. I usually denied their observation.

"How can a little girl look exactly like a grown man?" I'd say with my hands on my slender hips, unconsciously imitating my father's own determined stance.

But our physical resemblance and shared character traits were uncanny: long-armed, big-lipped, blue-eyed, loose-jointed, freckle-skinned, angst-ridden Bercaws. Except for our male and female chromosomes, nearly everything about us was a perfect match.

Yet I always felt like my own person. Even at a young age, I preferred stories to science. I wanted to write; Dad wanted to cure. We weren't exactly the same.

My dad, Dr. Beauregard Lee Bercaw, decided to become a neurologist after watching his father—the accidental curator of this gene pool—succumb to Alzheimer's. My dad feared that because he looked just like his dad, the disease would come for him, too.

So great was his worry that my dad the doctor even kept his father's autopsied brain in a jar on his office desk. Consequently, grandpa's gray matter and my dad's macabre dread became the center of my childhood universe.

"Use your head for something other than a hat rack," I heard repeatedly in my youth, because lazy thinking was the staunch enemy of any Bercaw. My dad hoped that he could ward off Alzheimer's by constantly trying to improve his mind, and mine. He paid me to read books one summer in high school when I asked if I could work at McDonald's.

I had my own Merck Manual by age ten. I learned the Heimlich maneuver from Dr. Heimlich himself. Meanwhile, my father busied himself with a second mortgage on our house to buy the first CT scanner in the state of Florida.

As my father approached middle age he began to experiment on himself with diet supplements. By age sixty he was taking seventy-eight tablets a day. He tracked down anything that offered the possibility of saving brain cells and killing free radicals: Omega 3s, 6s, 9s; vitamins E and C; ginkgo biloba, rosemary, and sage; folic acid; flaxseed.

This was 1999, mind you, long before herbal supplements were household words. My dad also eschewed sugar and alcohol. He played tennis three times a week. He scolded me when he saw sodium laureth sulfate listed as an ingredient in one of my shampoo bottles.

After retiring from his neurology practice, my dad turned his full attention to math puzzles. Even when I was visiting, he'd sit silently on his leather recliner with a calculator to verify the accuracy of computations he did by memory. I quietly wished that he would talk to me.

Be careful what you wish for, he had warned me many times. As if to clarify the point, Dad looked up from his *Sudoku* game once to say, "Promise me that you'll put a gun to my head if I turn out like my father."

I didn't kill my dad. Instead, I watched helplessly as he declined. He spent the last eighteen months of his life in a memory care facility until a Methicillin-resistant Staphylococcus aureus infection ravaged what was left of him.

My dad died on April 2, 2012, a month before his seventy-fourth birthday—the same age at which his own father had passed away.

I've been seeing a lot of my dad again lately. And not just in the mirror. He comes to mind whenever I forget to take my antidepressant medication. Or when a name escapes me. Worse yet, when I witness my nine-year-old son acting like a Bercaw.

I wonder what I might find if I could look behind my face into my brain. Amyloid-beta plaques settling into my shrinking cerebrum? Neurofibers tangled with tau protein? Proof I am the next Bercaw up to bat for Alzheimer's disease?

My father believed I was. For my thirty-fifth birthday, he surprised me with the genetic test for the APOE marker, which can indicate a predisposed genetic risk for Alzheimer's. APOE-2 is relatively rare and may even provide some protection against the disease. APOE-3 is the most common and appears to have a neutral role. APOE-4 indicates the highest risk factor.

Like my father, I carry the APOE-3 gene, which means I may or may not get the disease.

But he did get Alzheimer's—and he believed I would, too. Regardless of our indeterminate test results, he inferred that Bercaws and Alzheimer's were part of the same double helix.

Still, I can choose not to be like my father. I may have inherited his genes, but I can decide not to share his obsession. I don't want to spend the second half of my time on earth worrying about whether or not I'm going to get Alzheimer's disease.

I want to show my son what's worth living for—and the answer isn't math. Life is measured in love, not in brain mass.

~Nancy Stearns Bercaw

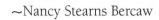

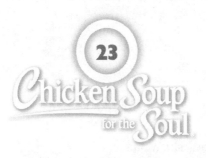

23

Managing with Mom

Laughter is the sun that drives winter from the human face.
~Victor Hugo

Every spring my Floridian in-laws returned to Michigan to visit their eight grown children, and my husband and I were first on the list. When they arrived in 1996, it didn't take long to notice my mother-in-law's memory was worsening.

My mother-in-law, who I called "Mom," was diagnosed with Alzheimer's at age sixty-five and prescribed a medication protocol to help manage her symptoms. The meds seemed to help, but over time, her memory lapses became more frequent and caused more concern. There were dinners burnt beyond recognition, repetitive stories and the constant struggle to remember names.

Then she came to stay with us one spring. It was difficult to find things for her to do around the house. I knew she loved working with plants and flowers, so pruning the dormant plants after our Michigan winter seemed a perfect fit.

I paraded Mom around the yard like she was some kind of master gardener with full control of her mental senses. "This can be cut back, but not this, this, and this." What was I thinking?

As I watched her work from the kitchen window, it was evident I needed a better plan.

The Japanese maple tree, yes, the one that had taken more than twelve years to grow to a mere four feet, was stripped to stubble. But I refused to let the disease have the upper hand.

Once again, Mom and I walked the perimeter of the yard, this time with a can of spray paint.

"Okay, Mom, cut back any plant sprayed with red paint. If you don't see red, don't cut."

"I can do that," she replied.

And it worked!

This was just the beginning of the many challenges Alzheimer's would bring to our family. There was the time Mom professionally cleaned my bathroom mirrors and glass shower doors with deodorizing spray. I watched as she worked intently to remove every self-induced streak. Occasionally she would tear a sheet from the roll of paper towel tucked under her arm. It was a brief "life as usual" moment for Mom; she felt useful and I didn't have the heart to stop her.

When a family member has Alzheimer's, you learn to laugh when you want to cry. Laughter becomes the healing balm for the isolation and loneliness we feel caused by our inability to communicate with someone we love. That 1996 visit with my mom-in-law was a precious gift.

I remember a long drive home from a family gathering with Mom seated next to my husband, Chris. The conversation went like this:

"Christopher, it is so nice to see you again." (10-minute pause)

"Christopher, it is so nice to see you again." (10-minute pause)

"Christopher, it is so nice to see you again." (5-minute pause)

That marathon conversation lasted two hours. It's now a cherished memory that makes us laugh every time we mention it.

I was surprised that the more time I spent with Mom, the more I longed to delve into the corrupted thought process of Alzheimer's disease. I spoke with home care nurses at the hospital where I worked. Many cared for those with Alzheimer's on a daily basis and their shared insight of the stages of the disease process was helpful. The Alzheimer's Association website (www.alz.org) and message boards were another great source of information.

For instance, I couldn't help but wonder what compelled someone to hide used paper placemats beneath the kitchen sink. When we would visit, Mom proudly displayed the food-stained placemats.

"Look, Christopher, I have been saving these for you. How many would you like?"

On our way out the door, they were discarded with the knowledge many more were sure to follow. If Mom wasn't gathering paper placemats from the dining tables at the extended care facility, she was stealing toilet paper from their public restroom. One Christmas, the family was invited to attend a sing-a-long in the community room at Mom's care facility. As my husband walked his mother back to her room he noted she was walking slower than usual.

"What's wrong, Mom? Are you tired?"

"Oh no, I'm fine."

As they rounded the corridor's corner, the two rolls of toilet paper hidden beneath Mom's sweater fell to the floor.

"What's going on, Mom? Are you lacking in toilet paper?"

"Well, I didn't want to accuse anyone," she replied, "but someone is stealing my toilet paper."

"Do you want me to report this to the front office?"

"Oh no," Mom responded, "I can get all the toilet paper I need from the public restroom next to the cafeteria."

We never knew what to expect when spending time with her and, looking back, it was laughter that helped us cope. We have no idea why she placed empty toilet paper rolls under her mattress, or why holding an infant brought clarity to Mom's confused mind. Sadly, the mystery of Alzheimer's disease is locked in the mind of those who suffer its debilitating effects.

It was difficult to watch Mom's sharp mind spiral downward. She had taught nursing at a well-known university and had given birth to eight healthy children, all who had graduate degrees and successful careers. Watching this once vibrant woman live in a world of void was heartbreaking.

My mother-in-law's life came to a quiet end as she watched her caregiver decorate the Christmas tree. I can only guess her thoughts in those last minutes before death.

Ultimately, I would like to believe God renewed her mind with flashbacks of all the amazing ways she touched the lives of her family and friends. Even as she failed, she continued to add value and be an important part of our family.

~Denise Marks

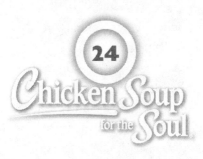

24

I Yelled at You Today

Patience is also a form of action.
~Auguste Rodin

I yelled at you today. I had gone to the kitchen to start dinner. What was I, twelve feet away? And you called out, "Where are you, where are you?"

"I'm right here in the kitchen," I answered angrily.

"Oh," you replied with a sigh of relief.

I yelled at you today. This time I was in the bathroom.

"Where'd ya go? Pat? Pat?" You called my name over and over.

"I'm in the bathroom," I shouted at the top of my voice, knowing full well you couldn't hear me, certain the neighbors could.

I yelled at you today. You poured apple juice on top of your pasta. God, what a mess.

I yelled at you today. You spit out your medicine. You'd never done that before.

I yelled at you today. You could see our car from the living room window and kept hinting for a ride. When I tried to explain that we had already been out, you looked at me as if I were trying to trick you. I hate it when you think I'm lying to you. Even though I know you can't help it, I hate it.

I yelled at you today. I had just finished dressing you for day care and left to answer the phone. When I got back, you had your nightgown back on and were wearing my oversized walking shoes. If that wasn't enough, when we were finally ready, as I zipped up your coat, you announced, "I have to pee."

At last, we were almost out the door. I put your favorite red hat on you. As I pulled it down over your ears, you smiled. "Thank you, Mama," you said and then instantly realized your mistake. You covered your mouth with your hand, your eyes wide with surprise. "That's what's happening, isn't it?" you asked.

"Yes," I answered. "And it's okay, it's okay," I repeated, trying to reassure us both.

But if it's okay, why can't I simply take the time to tell you I'm leaving the room and I'll be right back? Why yell when you make a mess at mealtime? I have to clean it up anyway. There are times when I can hardly get my own vitamins down; why do I always expect you to be able to swallow yours?

Tonight, as I tucked you in bed, we sang your favorite lullabies together. I think you enjoy this part of the day best. "I love you," I said and kissed you good night.

"I love you, too. How is it we're together?" you asked.

"Well, to begin with, you're my mother."

"Oh," you said, surprised. "Isn't that lovely?"

"It depends on how you look at it," I said, and you laughed. I thanked God you still had a sense of humor. "I'm sorry I yelled at you today," I apologized.

"You did?" you asked. But tonight that confused look was missing; instinctively I could tell you did remember.

"So, you're letting me off the hook," I said with relief. You reached up and moved the hair from my forehead.

"It's okay, honey, it's hard." And then you took the corner of your top sheet and wiped the tears from my eyes.

• • •

I didn't yell at you today. In fact, I haven't yelled at you all week. I'm finally taking the doctors' advice and the advice of family and friends. We won't be living together anymore. The guilt and grief is so overwhelming. I can hardly think straight. I'm tired, Mom, so very tired. After our ritual of nightly lullabies, I laid my head on your chest and sobbed like a baby. You cradled me in your arms and I knew you understood. Instantly, I began missing you more than I thought possible.

I visit you almost every day. Sometimes you remember my name, sometimes you don't. But you're always excited to see me. Today as I approached the dining room, your eyes were wandering, allowing me to sneak in and sit across the table from you. I waited for you to notice my presence. When you finally did, you smiled and asked, "Say, aren't you important to me?"

I got up from my chair and walked over to you. "I sure hope so," I said. After kissing you on top of your head, I added, "Because, God knows, you're important to me."

• • •

A year has passed; you've become weak and bedridden. Time for you is only a matter of days. The waiting is difficult. My two sisters and I are with you day and night. Today your favorite aides wait with us. I hold your hand and for the last time sing your favorite lullabies. "I'll be all right," I promise. "You can go now."

Your eyes close. Within minutes your breathing stops. The head nurse listens for a heartbeat. There is none. One of the aides walks over to the window. "We must free her spirit," she tells us, and, as is custom, opens it. Goodbye, Mom.

During our last few years together, I learned so much about you, so much about myself. Thank you, Mom, it was a pleasure. And an honor.

~Pat Tomlinson

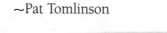

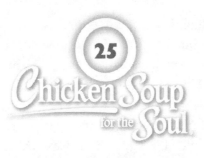

Fear and Self-Pity Are My Mortal Enemies

Never ask, "What reason do I have to be happy?" Instead ask,
"To what purpose can I attach my happiness?"
~Robert Brault, www.robertbrault.com

I am powerless over Alzheimer's. There is nothing I can do to change the fact that the man I love has this horrible disease. There is nothing I can do to slow the progression or alter the fact that his essence was lost to me so long ago. There is nothing I can do to change the fact that our life and our daughter's life will never be what he or she or I had dreamed.

This realization, the acceptance of the bitter truth, was a pivotal point for me. It marked the moment in my life when I made the decision to *live* with this disease and its effect on my world. I call this moment "coming out of the cave."

How I got to this point was through education and experience. The education gave me a scientific understanding of what I was dealing with, the legal and financial issues at hand, and the effect this disease and its inevitable progression would have on my immediate household. Unfortunately, the experience was the defeat I found at every turn early on. Denial and anger wouldn't make this disease go away. My depression only made it harder to cope. My bargaining with God or anyone else I hoped could change it was futile.

At first I was crushed. But then the challenge became clear: What was I to do to help my husband make his last chapter a grand finale? How would I nurture myself to maintain the physical, emotional, and intellectual strength to care for and provide for my family? How was I to guide our daughter, age three at the time of diagnosis, toward becoming a strong and capable young woman with as little baggage as possible? I don't know why, but I laugh as I write that part. I find it funny that early on I was so focused on getting rid of whatever would make her baggage too large a burden.

I'm not positive that I did it all in the best order, but I did it as it came to me, as the opportunities unfolded. And that day of my awakening, I also made the decision that I feel is the most important one of all. I decided to simply do my best. And, I decided that I would try with all my might not to judge the results of my efforts.

We built a fellowship. We connected with others affected by this disease. We shared our story with individuals and with groups. The effect was exhilarating. I have always said that when you share bad stuff it gets smaller and when you share good stuff it gets bigger. In Jay's face I saw a new level of comfort as he chatted with others who were also having difficulty speaking, remembering words, and organizing thoughts. He started to laugh more. I met some caregivers who were ahead of me, and in them I saw proof that survival was possible. In them I found new ways of coping. With them I found humor in the situations that previously infuriated me or pushed me to tears.

We helped others. In the people we met who were a bit behind us on this road we found proof that we were managing better. We found new self-esteem in guiding them and watching them grow. We accepted with true gratitude all opportunities to share, to help create or improve programs, to change legal roadblocks, or to raise awareness. We opened our hearts and made our struggle known so others would not feel shame in doing so, too. And privately we laughed about how hilarious it was that we got so much attention since all we knew was our own experience. My favorite memories of Jay are when he would joke about how little we knew and what would happen when everyone found out. But his knowledge that we had so little to offer never made him too afraid to accept an opportunity to give back.

We fine-tuned our faith. And I don't mean organized religion or spirituality. I mean the simple faith that everything happens for a reason. The faith that all is exactly as it should be. Our faith was multiplied by the coincidences we began to see around us. Like when I was buying a dress for an event, and I suddenly burst into tears. I explained to the dismayed salesperson that my husband had Alzheimer's, he was so young, and I was buying this dress to travel *without* him to an event. There I would be honored for my support of his efforts to make a difference. She stared at me in disbelief, and through tears told me her sister had been declining with what her family was beginning to believe was dementia. I was able to suggest a few resources to start with and then I bought the dress and we hugged goodbye. My trust that everything would be okay, that *we* would be okay, grew as random opportunities to give or receive support popped up. I saw that if my eyes were open to others, I would be shown the way to make it all work.

Lastly, I continually assess my attitude and behavior, looking for fear and self-pity. Fear paralyzes me and convinces me that I will not survive. That breeds self-pity, which blocks my ability to effectively solve the problems that arise. Self-pity makes me play the role of victim, which pushes me away from my family and friends, my critical support system. The more I fear and the more I pity myself, the more self-seeking I become in all my actions. Self-seeking causes behavior that negatively impacts my self-esteem. Poor self-esteem makes me depressed and tired. Fatigue affects my ability to do what I need to do, and fear pops up again. It all creates stress, and stress kills caregivers. It is a vicious cycle, hence my mantra that fear and self-pity are my mortal enemies.

So there you have it. I became aware of the truth. I accepted it for what it was. I chose to make the best of it in any way I saw available. And what did I get, honestly? I got the gift of self. The gift of an insight into what makes me happy. I didn't get my husband back, but I got myself.

~Laura Suihkonen Jones

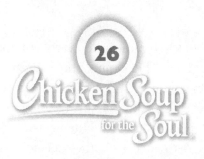

26

Sharing the Journey

Friendship is a sheltering tree.
~Samuel Taylor Coleridge

"This is such a hard journey," I thought, as I looked around the circle of caregivers gathered for our monthly support group. "What if I didn't have these friends to help me along the way?"

I exchanged brief smiles with the two women and one man who in the past year and a half had become three of my closest friends. One woman's mother had Alzheimer's. The other woman and the man cared for spouses with Alzheimer's like I did. As my husband Ray's confusion and anxiety increased, the road sometimes got so bumpy I felt I couldn't navigate it without these people.

When I first met Erika in a six-week Early Memory Loss Series offered by the Alzheimer's Association, I was immediately drawn to her. I noted the way she gently touched her mother on the shoulder and eased her into a chair, then sat beside her and took her hand. She was soft-spoken, with a broad smile for everyone and infectious enthusiasm for every topic that came up.

As the series progressed, I listened to Erika's excellent questions. They stimulated my own thinking. I'd read that caregivers often experience a sluggish mind because of the stress of the job, and I was no exception. I welcomed the intellectual stimulation she offered along with her example of kindness.

Erika and her mother began coming to our house for coffee

before an art class at the Alzheimer's Association. One morning she started talking about her work in the early childhood program at a community college near her home, and I jumped up to retrieve a copy of a book on parenting styles I had written two decades earlier. She held the book to her chest, her eyes shining.

"I love these theories," she said the next week as we sipped our coffee. "Come speak to my class at the college."

I shook my head. "I can't count on my brain to work."

"You'll be fine," she insisted.

Reluctantly, I agreed. As she introduced me to her class, I wondered if I could sort out and clearly explain ideas as I once had in workshops I taught. But when I began to speak, the ideas flowed.

"Thank you," I told her afterward, "for showing me I can still think."

I also met Marilyn and her husband in the Early Memory Loss Series. A lovely, silver-haired woman with sparkling blue eyes, Marilyn had a serene presence that literally awed me. I was anything but serene. "Don't you want to drive off a cliff sometimes?" I asked her one afternoon after class.

"Of course," she said with her tranquil smile. "Or push my husband off."

I laughed. Even Marilyn felt as frustrated as I did.

"When I feel like that, I focus on all the things we can still do together," she continued. "A hug. Dinner out. Going to a movie even if he can't follow all of it."

I thought of how I sometimes snapped at Ray when he asked the same question for the third time in five minutes, even though I knew he couldn't help it. I didn't want to be like that. I needed to be around Marilyn more.

We took a series of classes together, Powerful Tools for Caregivers, and afterward I plied her with questions about how she managed such a calm, peaceful demeanor.

She said it was her experience. She had been on this Alzheimer's journey three years longer than I had, and had once cared for a sister with special needs. She also went to Qigong several times a week, a

Chinese practice of aligning breath, movement, and awareness, and she regularly meditated.

Inspired to build more companionship into my days with Ray, I found that if I recorded television shows we both enjoyed, I could then pause them to answer his frequent questions, and rewind if I missed something while he talked. I hadn't watched much TV for years, but found we could enjoy many tension-free evenings that way.

When summer came I went to several Qigong classes that Marilyn helped teach, and I started meditating every evening. I still got overextended and anxious as Ray and I struggled with his capabilities, but I slowly developed more patience.

I met Milt at our adult community center's support group for caregivers of those with Alzheimer's. Every month I listened to this gracious man talk about his love for his wife and his unwavering commitment to care for her. Like Erika and Marilyn, he exuded an amazing warmth and kindness. Milt's wife and Ray shared some of the same aspects of Alzheimer's, but Milt sounded a lot more at peace with caregiving than I was.

Ray and I enjoyed both Milt and his wife, and the four of us began to meet regularly for coffee or lunch. We talked about the principle of "a day at a time"—how we needed to concentrate on the task at hand. While generally planning for the future, if we looked down the road too often, we overwhelmed ourselves with "what ifs," and couldn't do as good a job of solving current problems.

We talked of making sure we practiced gratitude for the things we had instead of stewing over the things that were no longer ours. And we grieved together. Our spouses couldn't do many of the things they had once enjoyed; the disease brought personality as well as physical changes, which affected our relationships.

I watched Milt take his wife's hand, or put an arm around her, and there was such tenderness in his actions that I wondered what the secret was behind his patience, understanding, and acceptance. Eventually I learned a deep faith in God sustained him. I had grown up in a religious family and believed in God and the power of prayer, but not with Milt's level of devotion. He was completely grounded in his love of the Lord.

Ray and I went to church several times with Milt and his wife, and afterward talked about the service over lunch. I had a hundred questions and he answered them, but never pushed his beliefs on me. Still, little by little, his influence seeped under my skin. I had experienced periods in my life when I felt close to God and turned to him often, but I wasn't in one of those times when Ray received his diagnosis. Slowly, following Milt's example, I found my way onto a more spiritual path. When my mood was grim, my patience short, I prayed for a quiet mind and peaceful heart, and was calmed and comforted.

Milt was speaking to the group now about how hard it was to watch his wife's decline. Erika and Marilyn nodded agreement. Who but these friends could truly understand what it is like to lose a loved one to this horrible disease? I took a deep breath. I could make this Alzheimer's journey, I thought to myself, because I had the example and support of these wonderful friends.

~Samantha Ducloux Waltz

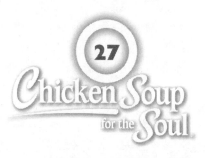

27

Where the Truth Lies

The greatest enemy of any one of our truths may be the rest of our truths.
~William James

My father doesn't know that my sister, Alice, is dead. He doesn't know that she had cancer, that she suffered, or that she, in a pain-pills-slur, asked to be buried in a red dress with no shoes.

My father doesn't know that I am his daughter, Elizabeth Emily, the girl he nicknamed "E.E." for brevity and affection. He thinks I'm my other sister, Valerie, because in his mind I am still twenty years old, not thirty. I am fifty pounds lighter, with a ponytail and head-phones. In his mind, I have never changed his diaper.

My father doesn't know he has Alzheimer's disease. He thinks it is 1964 and that he has just signed up for another tour in Vietnam. He's leaving tomorrow, so can we please stop worrying and press his uniform?

Some days, my father is not a man who needs Medicaid to share a nursing home room that barely fits three beds. He believes he is a California millionaire with so many servants and staff members he can't keep track of them.

There was a time I felt a naïve ethical duty to correct him.

You see, my father never lied to me. Not about Santa Claus or floating goldfish. Growing up, if I got caught in a fib, he'd gently warn: "Our Heavenly Father hates a liar." I knew from his steady example that my earthly father did, too.

So, when the most honest person I'd ever met started losing his grip on the truth I panicked.

I remember the first time his reality didn't match mine. He looked up from his hospital bed and asked, "Where's Tippi?" I froze. I couldn't remind him that he'd asked the vet to put his dog down three years ago. I couldn't lie, not to him, but I knew the truth would be painful, confusing, and cruel. Luckily, my husband piped up, "Tippi's in Texas." Technically, this was true.

Several times I tried to tell my father the "real" truth about things he'd say. "We sold the house in Tennessee ten years ago, remember?" I quickly found myself unintentionally hurting him.

I needed help learning how to give him back the very thing my "truth" and his Alzheimer's disease were taking—his dignity. In the worst moments of seeing him succumb to the disease, I prayed. My prayers were answered by a few heroic nurses who showed me the tools for maintaining dignity: patience, creativity, consideration, and love.

The first nurse, an unlikely baritone, harmonized "Que Sera, Sera" with my dad when he started belting out the song at 2 a.m. The nurse could have demanded that my dad quiet down, or worse, he could have medicated him. Instead, he sang a few choruses like they really were listening to old records, and his reassuring voice lulled my dad to sleep.

Another aide with a soft pink sweater taught me that sometimes a shrug, a warm smile, and a Hershey's Kiss provide more reassurance than anything we could say.

The best nurses taught me that when a loved one's mind deteriorates, you must talk to his or her heart. Though they taught me, they never told me. Their actions spoke to my heart and changed it as I witnessed the kindnesses they shared with all the residents.

I remember watching a favorite nurse ask one reluctant woman if she was ready to come downstairs for brunch. This puzzled me because the nursing home stood one-story high and it was 5 p.m. But it made sense to the woman. I later found out why she grinned and hurried toward the dining room. Her mother had called her "downstairs for brunch" every day in her youth and her mind had returned to those happy days.

Another tired afternoon I heard a different elderly woman cursing and screaming. A flustered new aide, in a rush to get everyone to supper on time, had wheeled her out of her room against her will. She fully believed that she'd been kidnapped. She scooted to the edge of her wheelchair seat and thrust both feet at the floor, slamming an imaginary brake. Her hands clutched a plastic baby doll with no shirt and wild hair. She shouted for the police, for a gun, for Jesus.

A wise older nurse ran up to her, smiling an authentic smile, and put some sugar in her voice, too: "Mama, the baby's hungry. Shall I take you to the kitchen and get her some milk?" The patient relaxed, nodded, and picked up her feet. She cradled her baby doll tightly and off they went with purpose, with dignity, with choice.

I once saw a beautiful young nurse let a gentleman believe she was his late wife. She blew him a kiss before she turned out his light.

Sometimes, my father thinks one of his nurses is one of us. He says, "Be good, honey. I love you." She replies, "I'll try. I love you, too!"

Now, when my father tells me he's a millionaire or that a dead loved one has stopped by for a pleasant chat, I am happy for him. I relax and smile. He relaxes and smiles back. Our hearts connect the same way they always have. His reality is every bit as real to him as mine is to me, and it is okay for me not to shatter the truths of his world.

Alzheimer's disease has tripped my father and sent him spiraling down a rabbit hole. His nurses have shown me that if I appear in a tree and tell him that this way is this and that way is that, he will simply lose his head. I have given up hope that, like Alice in Wonderland, he'll wake up from his surreal dream and come back to us. The nurses who have loved and cared for our entire family have helped me make peace with the fact that he is headed to the same place the other Alice, my sister, has gone. These heroic nurses have rushed around in scrubs and coats like White Rabbits. They have hurried between our world and the equally "real" places and times in their patients' minds.

I am grateful to these nurses for showing me the way through the darkness and chaos of my dad's dementia. I will be forever grateful to them for showing me my father's truth where it lies.

~Elizabeth Parker Garcia

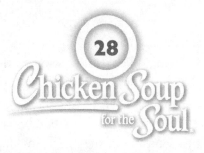

It's Sunday the 23rd

When life gives you a hundred reasons to cry, show life that you have a thousand reasons to smile.

~Author Unknown

D ad's face lit up as he opened the front door. "Jeri! Glenda! My girls! I'm so glad to see you." He ushered us inside. "It's Sunday the 23rd. There are clouds with fog and a chance of rain."

As always, the sound of The Weather Channel in the background greeted us as we entered the house. Starting every conversation with the date and weather forecast was Dad's way of showing us that he was aware of his surroundings. I often find myself waiting for him to announce the name of the current president and year, a result of too many memory tests and too many doctor's visits. All to prove he is alert and living in the present and that the diagnosis of Alzheimer's was wrong.

First came the constant drone of The Weather Channel. Next, small spiral notebooks that he tucked in his shirt pocket. Dad was constantly taking notes. More than a journal, it was a record of his day, his lifeline. What he did and when, who called, when they called, which visitors showed up, what they said, and what he said. Things he wanted to tell us, things he wanted to do. Notes he was constantly referring to throughout the day.

"I need help." With those words, he took the first of many steps down the slippery slope of Alzheimer's. He handed over his checkbook. "The numbers make no sense." He confessed that he had been trying to reconcile the bank statement for more than six hours and it was still off. Giving up control was so hard for my father. As a career Navy man, being in command was second nature. For the first time I saw tears in my father's eyes.

Once he was late coming home from his afternoon walk. A neighbor found him standing in the street, looking bewildered. He told her he had been looking for his house, but it was lost.

I don't remember the exact day I became the parent. One day I was coming to Dad for advice and information: "What's the recipe for Granny's sure-fire cough syrup?" I think it contained a slug of Jack Daniel's sipping whiskey. "How old was I when I broke my arm? How deep do you plant the tomatoes? Is it too late to trim the rose bush? Can you fix my bike?"

Then suddenly I was the one with the answers.

"It's time to replace the stove. The best buy is an electric one." No reason to tell him I was afraid the flames of the old gas stove would start a fire, or to mention the time gas filled the kitchen when the pilot light went out.

"The car's broken and we can't afford to fix it," I lied as I took away his keys. A ticket for driving too slowly on the highway, getting lost coming home from the corner store, backing into the mailbox; these things forced me to take away his independence. Being the parent meant making the tough decisions. It was a role no adult child should have to take on.

But not today. Sunday the 23rd was a good day for a visit. Dad was alert, happy, and content that his daughters were home.

As we settled on the couch, he suddenly stood up and went to his room. My sister and I exchanged questioning glances

Just as I was about to go looking for him, he returned with a smile. "How's your writing coming along? How's Larry's mother? Is Scott still driving a truck? Did you get a new puppy? Still liking your job at the library?" I was bombarded with questions about my family and pets.

Once again he disappeared, only to reappear in a few minutes.

This time it was my sister's turn to be questioned. She beamed as Dad asked about her husband and kids by name, mentioning details about their jobs and hobbies.

My curiosity got the best of me and I, too, made the trip down the hallway. What I found in my father's bedroom was astounding.

On the wall, above his desk, was a clothesline. On this line hung the important people in his life. There was a picture of me, my sister, brothers, relatives, next door neighbors, even the post lady. I couldn't even guess how he got the pictures, but there we were, looking like suspects in a police lineup.

Under each picture were our rap sheets, an index card with our names along with the names of our spouses, children, and grandchildren. Most touching were the lists of interests and dreams under each name. My father had come up with a unique way of holding onto his fading memories, a visual reminder of those he knew, loved, and interacted with.

I couldn't contain my admiration for him. He was fighting so hard to keep his world intact. He wasn't going to let his family slip away without fighting back.

I once asked my father what he considered his life's greatest achievements. "My family," he answered.

While Alzheimer's has robbed my father of many things, it has not robbed him of the love of his family and friends.

As my sister and I left that Sunday the 23rd, I realized that for a few hours, the fog had been chased away. The rain had not come. Dad knew our names.

~Jeri McBryde

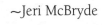

There is no one-size-fits all
formula when it comes to
Alzheimer's care. Needs change
at different stages of the disease
and each family's situation is
unique. Deciding on care can be a
tough decision.

"Care Options"
alz.org/care

Chapter 4

Living with Alzheimer's & Other Dementias

Next Steps and Tough Choices

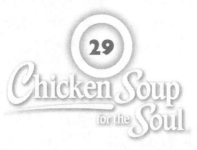

A Survival Guide for Alzheimer's Caregivers

The highest reward for a person's toil is not what they get for it,
but what they become by it.
~John Ruskin

t started innocently enough. A widower for more than forty years, my father began to struggle to find the right words and express himself. In time, he started repeating sentences and telling stories over and over again.

He was often confused and feared getting lost in the grocery store. Soon he did not recognize his favorite cereal box on the grocery store shelf, so he couldn't place it in his cart. He started to wear his pajamas over his clothes. He neglected to bathe and groom himself. His days and nights were mixed up. He would call me by the wrong name.

One night, while my father was still living alone, he called me.

"Jim, I'm so glad I reached you," he said. "I don't know where I am." I could hear the fear in his voice and it moved me.

"You're at home Dad—and you're safe," I assured him.

"No, I'm not in my house," he insisted.

"Dad, look at the address on the front of the house above the door. If it says 911, then you're in your home."

He set the phone down, picked up a flashlight and went out into the darkness to look at the house number. This was a weekly occurrence I had learned to solve.

He returned to the phone. "It says 911, but this is not my house. Will you please come over and give me a ride home?"

It was late and his home was on the other side of town. I tried my backup plan.

"Dad, look at the family pictures on the coffee table," I suggested. This technique worked every time. The photos reoriented him.

He set the phone down again and walked to the coffee table in the living room. When he returned to the phone I knew he had transitioned to the next stage of this disease.

"Did you look at the family pictures, Dad?"

"Yes."

"Well?"

"Jim, I don't know any of those people. Will you please come and take me home now?" I could hear the fear in his voice and remembered how he quelled my fear at age eleven when my mother died. He was an image of strength then. I needed to be that for him now.

"I'll be right over, Dad."

When I walked in the living room, he was waiting for me. "Please take me home, Jim."

"Okay, let's get you home."

Before I left the house, I turned on the front porch light. I backed out of the driveway and we drove to the corner. I turned right. I made three more right turns as I slowly drove around the block in the darkness. When we approached his house I asked him to look for his house number, 9-1-1.

When I pulled up in front of his house the front porch light was on.

"Can you see that house number, Dad?"

"9-1-1. That's it!" he said. I could sense his relief.

I walked him in to reorient him. He thanked me profusely; relieved to know he was home again.

As I started to return home I knew the time had come to admit him to an assisted living center.

My father spent several years in an assisted living facility for people with Alzheimer's. My siblings and I visited him nearly every day.

Alzheimer's is a long road for both the person with the disease and the family. Yet, I learned there is no higher honor than to serve a loved one during their time of greatest need. My father raised his six children alone. He did it with unconditional love, enviable patience, quiet strength, and an enduring sense of duty. It was our privilege to return the favor.

To care for someone with Alzheimer's you must be ready for the long haul. My five siblings and I learned how to cope and find hope in this arduous journey. Here is what we learned. I call them "The Ten R's." I think of them as a survival guide for Alzheimer's caregivers, and they may help you.

1. Reach out. After an Alzheimer's diagnosis, fear and uncertainty overwhelm you. To combat both, you need to reach out and get more information. Learn as much as you can, because knowledge is power. A deeper understanding of what you're up against not only helps you cope, but it also helps conquer fear. Contact the Alzheimer's Association in your area for seminars that will teach you valuable information to prepare you for this journey.

2. Rotate responsibility. Divide and conquer. If possible, share responsibility for caregiving with siblings or extended family members. The point is, don't carry this burden alone. If there are no siblings nearby, consider hiring a visiting nurse or senior's organization that specializes in home care. Two of my five siblings, Kathii and Joanie, along with her husband Ron, provided vital emotional support from their home across the country. Avoid isolation. You will need help, if not physically, emotionally.

3. Roll with the punches. People with Alzheimer's often make inaccurate statements as they draw from malfunctioning memory banks. Don't make the mistake I made and correct them. They will wear you out correcting you. Instead, roll with the punches.

4. Release your frustrations. Confide in a friend or another loved one. Alzheimer's is frustrating for everyone involved. Vent. Lean on

a friend. It's been said that friends multiply our joy and divide our sorrow. Share your pain.

5. Restore your perspective. Take a vacation. Find a way to get away from your caregiving routine. Easier said than done, but at least take a mini-vacation so you can restore your perspective, recalibrate your life, and come back refreshed and recommitted to the journey.

6. Remember who they "were." During the emotional strain and long course of care you can lose sight of who you're caring for. When I became exhausted, I could see my father as a needy old man. An angry old man. A forgetful and combative old man. If I could feel this way under duress, how would the caregivers at the Alzheimer's facility feel about him?

When my father's disease advanced to the stage where he had to be admitted to a specialized care facility, my five siblings and I set up a meeting with the entire staff of caregivers. The goal was to paint a picture of who my father "was" so they could appreciate who he "is." We shared photographs and stories of how he was the single parent of six children, a decorated Marine in World War II who fought at Iwo Jima, a cost accountant for the Chrysler Corporation, and a man so devoted to his wife and children that he never gave himself permission to remarry.

All six of his children painted a picture of who our father was—and who he is now. At the end of our presentation, the entire staff was in tears. Facility management later recommended that families admitting new residents introduce their loved ones to the staff in a similar way so they would "make a deep emotional connection with each new resident."

7. Rest. You must rest. This journey is long, hard, emotional, and exhausting. Find quiet moments to retreat and rest. Rest will restore your energy and, more importantly, your courage to tackle the next day. Listen to music, watch TV, or read. Reading a book like this one can help you recharge, relax, and feel less alone.

8. Rebound. If you make a mistake, learn to rebound. You are in uncharted waters. Your mistakes may irritate a loved one who is now prone to anger or combativeness. Accept mistakes and move on. Don't live with guilt if you admit your loved one to specialized nursing care before he or she is ready to go. They are never ready. And although they depend on you to make this call on their behalf, they may severely criticize you when you do.

When my father had to be admitted to an Alzheimer's facility, we decorated his room with familiar things and brought him there to visit for a few weeks. We told him this was his new apartment. Our hope was he would become comfortable and familiar with his room so when we moved him permanently it would not be traumatic for him and he would adjust quickly.

Our family selected the moving day together. We all had a role to play. My brother, Bob, took him out to lunch. Mary, Chris and his wife Sue, and I pulled up with a trailer and loaded his bedroom furniture and enough belongings to fit in the single room. We hung his pictures and set up his furniture. Bob brought him to the facility a few hours later. My father's reaction? He was furious. He looked at me, insinuated that he had been deceived and accused me of being the "ringleader." My throat tightened when he suggested that I betrayed him.

My father and I were very close all my life, so for him to feel I betrayed him cut me to the core. It was times like these I reminded myself that my father's accusations were "the disease talking." During this journey it is important to know the difference between when your loved one is talking and the disease is talking.

My father was a wise man and put his end-of-life instructions to me in writing when he was of sound mind so I would never second-guess myself if his verbal instructions contradicted his written instructions.

9. Rejoice. This is the most important "R." Rejoice in the privilege of serving your loved ones in their hours of greatest need. Abraham Lincoln once said of those who died in the Civil War, "... they gave

the last full measure of their devotion...." My father has been gone for five years and I can say with confidence that the six children he raised alone "gave the last full measure of their devotion" in caring for him as he faded from this life. Even when he took his last breath, Bob held his right hand and I held his left. And Bob's wife Patti, and my wife Karen, stood by us until the end.

10. Reflect. When your loved ones pass, take time to reflect on their lives. Even if you did not have a great relationship with them, reflect on the good times and how you faithfully served them.

Along with my siblings, we consider it a joy to have served our father until his death and we enjoy reflecting on his life of integrity and its impact on our children and us.

And isn't having a powerful and positive impact on others what life and legacy are all about?

~James C. Magruder

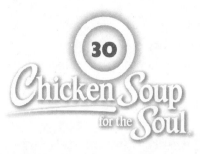

30

We Are a Family

Call it a clan, call it a network, call it a tribe, call it a family.
Whatever you call it, whoever you are, you need one.
~Jane Howard

Choosing between a skilled care facility and caring for a loved one at home is a difficult, and personal, decision. There are pros and cons no matter which choice you make. And there will always be someone around to let you know you made the wrong one.

I made the decision to put my mother into the care of professionals who are trained to handle the complexities of Alzheimer's disease. Did I have doubts about my decision? Almost every day. Did I think I could do a better job? Sometimes. Did I know that she was in a good place? Always. I knew she was safe, well fed, and well cared for. Those were the most important parts of the decision.

But what came as a surprise was the extended family I gained—the staff, other residents, and their families.

The observant staff can tell when I need a hug, or a few minutes of real conversation unrelated to Alzheimer's. And they're there when I need a shoulder to cry on.

The residents brighten my day by greeting me with big smiles and waves. I know they are happy to see me and I'm thrilled that my visit to my mother can bring so much joy to so many others. But I think I'm actually the lucky one, since my day just got better because they are all so happy to see me.

One resident always offers me a cup of coffee, having "just made a fresh pot." Another always asks if I would like a ham sandwich. If I am there at dinnertime, another asks if I would like something to eat, because she "made plenty."

All the visiting families bond, share stories, and help each other through the tougher days. We are there to share and support one another whenever needed, especially as a loved one's days draw to an end.

One family member still visits regularly, even though her mother passed away quite some time ago. Her visits are a gift to everyone. She made a huge impact on me one particularly difficult day when she got my mother to sing with her. "You Are My Sunshine" had been Mom's "go to" song in recent years, calming her down or bringing her out of a deep empty space. During the early days of her final stage of Alzheimer's, the dark unresponsive days were the hardest. I couldn't reach her. But when our newest family member came in and said, "Virginia, I want you to sing with me," Mom opened her eyes, smiled and sang "You are my sunshine, my only sunshine." She sang every word to all the verses.

There is no timeline to this disease. My mother has been in the final stage for more than a year now. I have witnessed others who have gone much more quickly, as well as those who seem to just keep moving forward at their own pace. Still able to play games, and do group activities. Still able to recognize me as a friend or an extended family member.

My mother's roommate lets me know what Mom has or hasn't done since my previous visit. She lets me know who has visited. And I have gotten to know most of her children. When our mothers are sleeping, we share stories. One of the daughters lives in Wyoming, and I see and talk to her more than I do members of my own family!

Choosing a skilled care facility can be a difficult decision, but it can also be heartwarming and rewarding, too. My new extended family truly understands what each of us is going through… together.

~Carolyn Mers

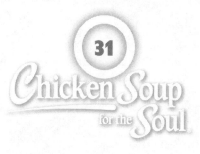

31

Yes, But I Still Know Him

The future is called "perhaps," which is the only possible thing to call the future. And the only important thing is not to allow that to scare you.
~Tennessee Williams

"I am sorry to say that Mr. Gunnett has mild cognitive impairment," the neurologist said matter-of-factly about my husband. "He is weak in certain areas of problem solving and cognitive reasoning."

That wasn't so bad, I thought, not knowing what the words meant. My resistance to what was coming helped me rationalize that everyone has memory loss as they age.

Our lives went along fairly smoothly for the next few years, until I started noticing Bob was forgetting more and more.

Again, I rationalized. It was his hearing loss. After all, how could he remember what I said if he couldn't hear it in the first place?

Life went on. He sang in a men's group, entertaining residents at nursing homes and worshipers in local congregations.

But now the time has come. I'm forced to accept that my husband has dementia, probably early-stage Alzheimer's. It saddens me to see his shop tools lying idle, when they used to hum along as he built project after project. His sense of melody is fading, too, and after many years singing praises to God, Bob's voice no longer harmonizes with his friends.

We are learning we can focus on the positive and cherish each day.

My friend Carisa recently reminded me: "Patty, it will be fine as long as he remembers he loves you," which he does.

For many years, I thought I could change Bob, or fix things about him, even the memory loss. Once I read a story about a preacher who surveyed 100 church members, asking them to write down what or who they would like to change. A pretty high percentage admitted they wanted to change their spouses, their bosses, their friends or family members. The preacher was dismayed that not one person said, "Change me."

Every day, I ask God to change me. I still have a way to go, but I pray for patience as Bob asks me the same question five times in five minutes. I empathize with his frustration at losing his memory, as I know it is beyond his control. And I pray a cure is discovered soon for this terrible disease.

On November 1, 2013, Bob went to live at Arden Courts memory care center as his memory deteriorated quite rapidly over the summer. It was an agonizing decision to make but I had to let go of what I wanted and realize what was best for him. He is well taken care of, plus God has continued to have him use his gift of singing to entertain the other residents, visitors and caregivers!

There is a story about a husband who visits his wife, who has Alzheimer's, in a nursing home. "Why do you visit her every day? She doesn't even know who you are," his friend says. "Yes, but I still know her," he replies.

For now, Bob still remembers who I am. But if the time comes when he doesn't, at least I can say, "Yes, but I still know him."

~Patty Gunnett

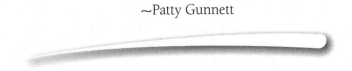

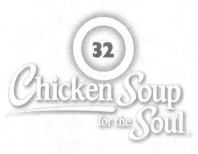

32

One Moment at a Time

Once you make a decision, the universe conspires to make it happen.
~Ralph Waldo Emerson

Pops, my stepdad, once flew stunt planes upside down, in dizzying directions, a hobby as confusing to others as his life must seem to him now that he has dementia.

"Where could your mother be this late?" he says, looking at me and frowning.

He scratches his chin stubble and shuffles in his slippers to the kitchen to prepare his dinner. He doesn't remember that Mom was in the intensive care unit and I had been with her for three days. He doesn't remember visiting her. He isn't too keen on my hanging out at their house each evening, either.

"You hungry? I'll fix you some chicken and potatoes, those cheesy ones you like," I offer.

"No thank you; I don't eat cheesy potatoes. I'll fix my own food."

He spreads peanut butter on crackers, and then chomps a handful of M&Ms. He sinks down on the sofa but can't get back up five minutes later. So I help him, the once strapping Navy man who wants to go to bed. He sits on the edge of his bed and waits for me to leave. Fifteen minutes later I see he's asleep on top of the covers, fully clothed. I return to the hospital to be with Mom.

In the morning I drive bleary-eyed to Pops' house to make breakfast. He is still asleep. I have to figure out what to do. I gaze at the framed family photographs and Mom's collection of ceramic angels.

I stare at the thermostat my parents adjusted frequently, regardless of the season. I cry quietly and curl up on the sofa in the exact spot Mom had slept in. I lay my head on her pillow and wait for Pops to wake up so I can tell him that his wife of fifty years has passed away.

After gently breaking the news, I ask, "Does your heart ache?"

"No. I'm thankful for all the time we had," he says in a moment of clarity. "My heart doesn't hurt. My ankle hurts."

I raise his pant leg and see a massive infection he developed from scratching a minor wound. The visiting nurse arrives, and tells me Pops can't be left alone. I agree to stay, never mind the funeral arrangements.

Pops is exhausted from answering the nurse's six-page questionnaire, and after she dresses his wound he goes back to bed.

When he wakes up he asks, "Where could your mother be? Why isn't she coming home?"

I know he's thinking, "And why are you still here?"

I can't cope alone another minute. When Pops starts snoring, I call my stepbrother who lives out of town and tell him I'll make the funeral arrangements for my mom. He'll make the arrangements for Pops' care.

My heart aches as I pack Pops' meager belongings: Bible, magnifying glass, favorite deck of cards for solitaire, and personal-care items. I fold his pants and remove his favorite chambray shirts from hangers. He watches, confused and irritated as I stuff his clean clothes into the wicker laundry basket.

"I'll carry that dirty laundry down the hall and do my own clothes," he says in a huff.

I stall him until my stepbrother arrives. His son coaxes him.

"Dad, the doctor says you can't stay by yourself because of your leg. There's a facility a block away from my house. You need to be there for a while. And I'll come see you every day."

Pops' face brightens; then he looks confused. I turn my head, cringing with heartbreak and guilt. Resigned, he nods. "Okay, I'll go for a little while."

Then he looks at me, "Where's your mother?"

I swallow the lump in my throat and tell him again. He nods.

Stoic, and satisfied for the moment, he follows us into the hall and locks the apartment door.

We dash through the rain to the car. I carry his things in a cardboard box, and my stepbrother carries Pops' clothes in the laundry basket. I lean in, hug him goodbye, and tell him I have a surprise for him. And I drop a forty-eight snack-pack box of M&Ms on his lap. He smiles broadly.

"I'll see you soon," I promise. Rain washes the tears from my face. I wave as he and my stepbrother drive off in a thunderstorm with lightning streaking the sky. I do my bést to take a deep breath, but can't seem to pull in enough air.

A few days after Mom's funeral, my stepbrother calls. "You won't believe this, but Dad has settled in. He eats breakfast, lunch, and dinner at the facility. He's even talking to the nurses and his tablemates. He flipped out his pilot's license at dinner and told them he's still a good-looking Navy man."

I laugh aloud. As difficult as the decision had been, Pops requires more long-term care than either of us can provide.

While I dismantle my parents' household, Pops and his son reconnect and spend time talking about old times. With better nutrition, hydration, and mental stimulation Pops stays awake longer. He becomes more sociable. I send him letters, cards, and photographs of him with Mom.

The way my stepbrother and I handle decisions about our parents' final days is probably the same way they handled our earliest days: overwhelmed, uncertain, and guilt-ridden.

I'm sure when my brother and I were babies, crying inconsolably, our parents' tears mingled with ours. As they cuddled us and sang lullabies, they must have felt uncertainty, too. When they looked into our faces, imagining our futures, they must have wondered how their actions would affect us.

The best any of us can do with loved ones who have dementia is to comfort and nurture them through all the stages. Lullabies aren't just for babies. We must sing. We must soothe. And we must take each day one moment at a time.

~Linda O'Connell

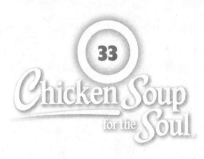

The Next New Step

What is a mom but the sunshine of our days and the north star of our nights.
~Robert Brault, www.robertbrault.com

I barely pulled off the road before the tears spilled onto my steering wheel. I turned off the engine and finally sobbed the long, panting, private sobs of despair that I had been holding deep inside me. I had just left my mother at her new home in an Alzheimer's care facility.

I found myself talking with my mother in my imagination. "Oh Mom, you held me when I broke up with my boyfriend and cried through the night. You took me from store to store to store to find the perfect prom dress. You went to all of my concerts, helped me fill out college applications into the night, and gave me advice on the curtains for my first house. I helped you find a new apartment after the divorce, and later had lunch with you at the new office you were so proud of. Together, we got lost driving, worried about whether Thanksgiving dinner would come out right, created homemade Christmas cards, and cried through my wedding. You cared for me when my first baby wouldn't stop crying. And now, today, we cry separately. And that is what hurts most."

After a while, the sobs quieter, I realized that I couldn't sit forever in a car full of tears by the side of the road. So I slowly put the car into gear and drove home.

The next day I went to visit Mom in her new place and found her happily folding napkins. I sat down to join in, privately thinking how sad it was that we were reduced to napkin folding. But, fold-by-fold, we watched a neat pile of smoothed napkins growing between us. She seemed okay with it all, and I found some of my own tension lifted when I left that day.

"Thanks for a good day, Mom," I thought, as I punched the numbers into the security lock to go outside.

A few weeks later, I thought it worth a try to go ice skating. Someone had said that activities from childhood were good for those with dementia, and she had loved to ice skate. I was not hopeful, thinking of the balance involved, the cold, the new-ness, and the frustration of wrestling into tightly laced skates. Leaving for the rink, I noticed she had mismatched shoes and I groaned inside. This was probably a mistake.

Later, after lacing up the skates and hiding her shoes under a bench, I helped Mom gingerly step onto the rink, and then she was in front of me skating and laughing. I couldn't help a few familiar tears as I watched her remember her way across the ice. She turned and caught me crying, then skated on.

"Thanks for the wonderful day," I said when we were done skating.

Slowly, I learned what worked and what didn't. A trip to the store made a lovely afternoon, especially if we stopped for ice cream. I began to notice that the pressure of trying to think of new and interesting things to do was going away. Nothing earth-shaking was required; it was good to simply sit and eat ice cream or walk through a garden. Each day Mom stopped at more or less the same place and noticed the flowers in bloom and the birds flying by. Soon I did, too.

Later, when Mom was unable to leave her room, I found it best to just sit by her side, without trying to talk. We listened together to the pleasant sounds around us and when it was time to leave, it was a simple "Bye, Mom, thanks" that completed the day.

And so it was that the world I had mourned so deeply that day in my car was replaced with a new world—a world that Mom owned, controlled, and embraced, once I gave her the chance. And then, magically, it was a world she allowed me to enter with her after

I let go of my own tangled expectations and let her show me how it was done.

It was a world with lovely flowers to smell and smooth, graceful napkins piling up into a beautiful stack. It was a world of quiet, gentle walks, delight in the adventure of a trip to the grocery store, a world where mismatched shoes do not matter, and an afternoon on ice skates was all we needed on our agenda. In her world, she showed me the beauty of the quiet and the completeness of two chairs side by side.

Oh Mom, you held me and helped me when I was small and when you were the grown-up. Now, just when I thought it was my turn to be the grown-up, you have showed me yet again how it is done. It should be no surprise that one thing has not changed at all — it was you who took my hand to show me how to take the next, new step.

Thanks, Mom, for all the wonderful days, then and now.

~Jennifer Harrington

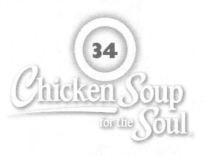

Shopping for Nursing Homes

If we are facing in the right direction, all we have to do is keep on walking.
~Buddhist Saying

As a teacher, I was grateful summer vacation had arrived so I could concentrate more on caring for my mother, who was approaching the middle stage of Alzheimer's.

Each day presented new challenges. I noticed Mom was losing track of time. She didn't know how to make her lunch or tell me if she had eaten. These moments made it clear that when I returned to school she would need someone with her.

I heard that a friend's former babysitter, Lula, might be available. I called Lula and she agreed to come two or three times a week so Mom would be comfortable with her when I went back to work. At first Mom was resistant to having someone there, but I knew she would be much happier being in her own home. I could not imagine my mother agreeing to go to a senior center or to adult day care.

At the same time, I began attending an Alzheimer's support group. At one meeting, someone said nursing homes sometimes had two-year waiting lists. I had found a temporary solution for day care, but I knew I needed to look ahead. One of the other group members and I decided to meet twice a week to visit nursing homes.

What an educational experience that turned out to be! I learned about the levels of assisted care, private pay, and Medicare. After several investigative trips, I placed my mother on two waiting lists, hoping I would never need them. My ultimate choice in homes was one where I saw reading materials displayed in all the common areas. During mealtimes, residents with dementia were seated with other residents. My thought was that if residents with dementia were always kept together, their skills would decline more quickly, whereas if they were with other talkative people, even if they had difficulty joining in, they could listen and help keep their minds alert.

My mother that summer kept asking me why I would not take her out with me. We usually went everywhere together, even if it was just to have the oil changed in the car. I am a terrible liar and coming up with excuses was getting harder and harder. I felt worse each time I fabricated a story.

One evening when she was especially lucid, I sat with her and told her how much I loved her and how I wanted to take care of her. She had to let Lula come so I could go to work. Then, I don't know where the courage came from, but I did something I have never regretted. I told her that I would keep her home with me as long as it was humanly possible, but someday she might have to go into a nursing home for the best care possible. We both cried and I asked her to trust me.

I did not tell her this for her sake, but for mine. If the time came when she needed to live in a nursing home, I knew she might not be mentally aware of the situation. I was asking permission and forgiveness in advance, and gratefully, I received them.

~Jean Ferratier

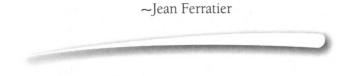

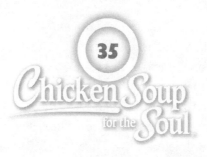

No Matter What

Painful though parting be, I bow to you as I see you off to distant clouds.
~Emperor Saga

Fall 2013

My mother's journey was not an easy one. She did not pass through the beginning and middle stages of Alzheimer's gently. Confusion and mood swings were mixed with obsessive compulsions — such as counting change. Conversations were misunderstood and lead to volatile situations, or there were fleeting moments of lucidness when I knew I had my mom and she knew me as her child. Those moments few and far between.

Eventually there was just silence. Did a small part of who she was still exist? I'll never be sure, but what I know and say to others when asked, is just remember that you love them and want them to know that, no matter what.

Spring 1997

My mother sits at the dining room table, her morning ritual underway. Silently I watch her. Her purse and its contents are splayed on the dark wood surface.

Her focus this morning is on the loose change in front of her. A pencil and paper lie beside her wallet. She is counting out loud. One hand pushes the change around on the table's surface as she counts.

"Two times five is ten. I have one… two… three… four… five! Five 25-cent pieces."

She starts to write the amount down.

"That's five times twenty-five… but I also have pennies over here. I'll start again… one… two… three…"

Along with the separated groups of coins are the beginnings of a pile of crumpled pieces of paper. Each piece of paper has crossed out, written-over, pencil-scrawled additions, sometimes with two or three partial or completed sums. Those sums will neither answer nor satisfy my mother's need to count.

"There…" she says, looking at me, putting the pencil down, "that's done." And then a slight frown. "I think I should count it again. I'm sure I had more."

This morning I don't offer to help. I decide to make breakfast.

"Wendy…"

I push the button to start our morning coffee and turn to see my mother walking toward me. Her hand reaches up to touch my face. She speaks to me in those next few moments as my mom. The veil of Alzheimer's temporarily lifted.

"I want you to know this. You are my daughter, my baby. I love you. Don't ever forget that."

We hug each other. "I love you too, Mum. Always, no matter what."

Then the knowing flash ends. I see it in her eyes, then her face. My mother goes back to the dining room table to recount her change. I butter the toast and pour coffee for our breakfast.

Fall 1999

We walk up and down the hall, stopping at each cheaply framed painting decorating the otherwise barren hallway. My mother reviews each piece. Her comments have varied little over the last few months.

We stand in front of the locked door that allows visitors and staff in and out. She looks at the keypad.

"Lots of numbers. People play with them sometimes."

We continue our walk.

"June," says a voice from the nurse's station, "you have a visitor today." I don't recognize the staff member. She must be new.

"Yes," my mother says, "this is my sister." I smile. Well, at least I am still a member of the family.

The nurse introduces herself, adding, "I take it you are the daughter?"

"Today, just happy to be my mother's sister."

The nurse smiles. "Good for you."

My mother and I continue our walk. The sunroom is ahead of us. "Shall we sit down, Mum?"

We only sit for a minute or two. She is restless and needs to move. Once again, arm-in-arm, we continue our walk, stopping to look at cheap paintings that hang on otherwise barren hallway walls.

Winter 2001

I lean over the slightly raised bed railing. Our faces inches apart. My lips kiss her cheek. "How are you today, Mum?" I smile. A flicker of a smile softens her thin angular face. It is an automatic response to an automatic question. My mother is still polite — but her eyes tell the truth.

Her colour is good but she is thin, far below her normal weight, and she looks so fragile. My hand touches her gray and thinning hair. I lift it gently upwards. It feels clean and soft. Then I watch the strands of hair as they fall, not quite back in place, but not out of place either. I repeat this motion again and again. "When I was a child," I say out loud, "you used to do the same thing."

Silence.

I take her hands in mine. So warm. Soft. Our fingers explore the protruding veins on top of each other's aging hands.

The bed rail digs into my rib cage. I raise myself up slightly. Leaning over again I reposition myself closer so she can hear me.

"Your name," I begin, "is June." My words are practiced and my speaking voice low. The narrative is always the same.

"Your name is June Charlien Carmen Card. Your maiden name was June Charlien Carmen Loucks."

Her hazel eyes watch me. I think that perhaps today she is listening to my voice. I continue telling my mother about the life she lived, a life she herself had often talked about.

"Your husband's name was Lorne."

I feel my back spasm slightly from the strain of leaning over the bed rail. I try not to finish too quickly.

"You had a baby girl. I am that girl." I smile at her, and continue, "I am your daughter. My name is Wendy.

"Your name is June. I am your daughter."

My practiced words end. I stand up stretching my back. Her hazel eyes stare at my face. I hope she will just once more say my name, just once more soften the stare and give a smile of recognition. There is no acknowledgment.

Then her body turns slightly away from me and she closes her eyes. Like a child does when ready to sleep after the bedtime story has been told.

"And," I add, leaning forward one last time, "I love you very much. No matter what."

~Wendy Poole

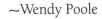

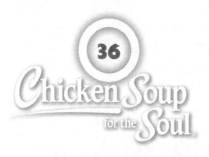

Songs of Remembrance

Music washes away from the soul the dust of everyday life.
~Berthold Auerbach

My mother was diagnosed with Alzheimer's disease in 2011, but her condition didn't progress quickly until she lost her first child, my oldest sister Mary Ann, to colon cancer. At that time, despite excellent medical and moral support, the disease progressed rapidly.

Right now she is still living in her own home in Massachusetts, with constant care from my siblings and her grandchildren who live nearby. The siblings like me who live farther away are regularly scheduled to provide respite. I live about three hours away by car and my opportunity to care for our mother comes every third Monday for twenty-four hours. I use the word "opportunity" because as one of twelve children, I feel blessed and privileged to attend to this wonderful woman who so influenced my life.

But despite being an adult with a family of my own and a whole congregation who look to me for comfort and leadership, I miss my mom. I am accustomed to her being a source of wisdom, joy, and encouragement in my life. At this point I find myself in deep need of all three. Last year I not only lost Mary Ann, who was like a second mother to me, but I also lost four dear friends, and had neighbors who passed on as well.

Then, just months later, I experienced one of the most horrific tragedies of our time, as I live and serve in Newtown, Connecticut.

The unfathomable losses involved in the Sandy Hook Elementary School massacre have deeply affected hundreds of people I love, including my two young children who attend public school in the same town. Before, in times of difficulty, my mother was the person I could always turn to for guidance and comfort.

Recently, as I made the long drive to my mother's home, I found myself praying to God: "Dear Lord, would you please show me a sign of your Spirit still at work in her life and your joy still emanating from her heart? I am in deep need of encouragement."

That day, our time together seemed about as routine as it could be. When I picked her up to take her to the hairdresser she asked the usual questions about who I was and where we were going. She also asked, as she does frequently, whether or not I am married and have any children. (My wife and daughters were the happy recipients of my mother's love in the years prior to Alzheimer's.)

Later, as we drove along to run a few more errands, I looked over at her while at a red light and noticed she had completely zoned out. I could tell she was unaware and oblivious to her surroundings. I felt so disheartened. But then I had a flashback from when I was six years old in a summer camp run by our Catholic church. My mother volunteered there and she led a lot of singing. I recalled something I had read in one of the many helpful books from the Alzheimer's Association: People with Alzheimer's often won't remember recent conversations, but they will remember old songs. While I was driving, one of the songs my mother taught me at that camp nearly forty years ago popped into my mind:

Thank You Lord for giving us love,
Thank You Lord for giving us love,
Thank You Lord for giving us love, right where we are.
Alleluia, praise The Lord.
Alleluia, praise The Lord.
Alleluia, Praise The Lord, right where we are!

The words of this song came tumbling out of my mouth as I sang out loud in my car. My mother's eyes lit up and she woke from her daze. Then she began to sing. She not only remembered the tune, but all the lyrics, too. She didn't miss a beat.

We wound up singing several songs from that long ago camp. She praised Our Savior in whose spirit we sang. Her voice was so loud that I could have sworn the kids in the car next to ours were joining the chorus. I was flooded with joy for this moment that was musical and magical.

At last, when our singing subsided, this lovely lady sighed, looked at me, and asked, "Who taught you these songs?"

I responded, "My mother did."

She took a deep breath and exclaimed, "Your mother must be a very wonderful woman! I'm sure I would love her if I knew her!"

I chuckled at this and said, "She still is and you sure would!"

I felt I had my mom back then. Even more importantly, I knew my Father in Heaven had answered my prayer for my mother on earth. It was the best gift I could have received during this season of my soul.

~Jim Solomon

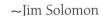

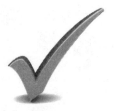

Be realistic. The care you give does make a difference, but many behaviors can't be controlled. Grieve the losses, focus on positive times as they arise, and enjoy good memories.

"Five tips to help you cope"
alz.org/care

Living with Alzheimer's & Other Dementias

Taking the Journey with Your Parent

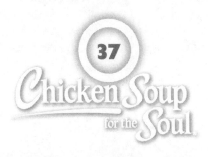

Feeding Squirrels with Dad

Tension is who you think you should be. Relaxation is who you are.
~Chinese Proverb

Every Wednesday, as I have for the past two years, I leave work and drive to the nearest fast food restaurant. I order a strawberry milkshake and make the twenty-five-mile trip to visit my dad, who has dementia and lives in a nursing home. The routine is familiar—parking, walking up the winding driveway, entering the tastefully decorated lobby and signing in with the receptionist. Then it's a right-hand turn down the long hall to the wing where my father lives.

Dad won't be in his room when I arrive. Members, as the residents are called, aren't in their private rooms except to sleep. They are encouraged to be involved with one another and to participate in activities throughout the day.

As soon as I pass through the arches of the doorway I spot him. The aides that care for my father are angels. My father looks as he would at home—in casual slacks and a T-shirt or sweater, he is well groomed. Most days he also wears one of his beloved baseball caps. Usually it's the red one that proclaims "My grandson is a U.S. Marine." He has no idea which grandson the hat refers to, and if asked will usually tell a big tale of his time in the Marines (he was never in the military).

Within seconds his head twists around, his hand comes up in a wave, and a smile lights up his face as he spots me. My father doesn't know what he had for lunch; he doesn't know what year or month it is, but he knows who I am and he's always happy to see me.

I reach his side and hand him the milkshake. We exchange the same greeting every week.

Dad says, "How did you know where to find me?"

I always respond, "Mom told me."

As we wheel down the hall toward the main entrance he eagerly begins to drink his milkshake, telling me that strawberry is his favorite, and asking how I knew. On our way out the door, we pass staff members, other visitors, and members. All of them, and I mean every single one, smiles and greets my father by name. Even now, he is the man everyone knows and loves. Sometimes they will touch my shoulder and say, "Your father is such a delight."

The facility has immaculate lawns with flower gardens and private areas for visitors to sit and spend time with their loved one. In my father's previous world, as I refer to it before dementia, he loved roses. So our favorite place is the rose garden. As we make our way there, he will usually ask if I want him to push the wheelchair because it's a lot of work. I smile and assure him that I can use the exercise. We stop and I pull up a chair and settle in; he is drinking his milkshake as I am catching my breath.

When my father became a resident of the nursing home, I was in the midst of my busy life. My middle son had been deployed to Iraq. I constantly worried about him, and I had two other sons still at home. I have a full-time job, a house, a husband, volunteer activities, and the same list of responsibilities as most busy women. There are a lot of Wednesdays when the workday ends and all I want to do is go home. I want to get dinner on the table, get my chores done, and try to squeeze in an hour of relaxing with my husband before going to bed and getting up and starting all over again. But I can't. Because it's Wednesday and the responsibility I feel to make sure Dad has a visit weighs on me.

Once I'm with him, my mood lifts. When we sit in the garden a sense of peace comes over me. The rest of the world doesn't exist as we talk about the same things over and over or sit quietly together. I'm forced to set aside the rest of my life. I'm forced to be "in the moment." In this day and age when all of us multitask to accomplish as much as we possibly can in twenty-four hours, it's a rare treat to be this calm.

Sometimes it hits me that five years ago Dad had the same life most of us do. He was up before the sun and exhausted every night trying to get it all done. But then one morning, he woke up and that life ceased to exist. Dementia had taken its hold.

Now we sit in the rose garden and talk about how he "built" the building behind us. We talk about the weather, the trees, the roses, and whether he slept well last night. Ten minutes from now, we will talk about the exact same things, except it will all be brand new to him.

Soon, if we are quiet enough, the real reason we are here in this garden appears. Our special guests begin to arrive. One by one, their little legs carry them to a cautious spot not too far from us but not too close, either. Their beady black eyes and big bushy tails might turn some people off, but not us. I pull the bag of peanuts from my purse.

"Look, Daddy." I point out their arrival as if I'm five years old, but now it's my father who is childlike. I take the empty milkshake cup from him and hand him a bunch of peanuts. Slowly he tosses the first one to the closest squirrel, who eagerly snaps it up and stands on his hind legs to peel it. Dad grins and turns his focus to the next squirrel. Over and over he tosses peanuts to squirrels of all colors and sizes. One is missing half his tail, which prompts a weekly conversation about how we think he lost it. Sometimes a few chipmunks will show up, but mostly it's the squirrels who, through some unspoken squirrel underground, have found out there are peanuts to be had.

Dad smiles at their antics and tells me for the sixth time in an hour that he loves "those little guys." I smile and agree that squirrels are wonderful.

In his other life my father was able to coax squirrels to eat from his hand. Dad never made a ton of money, he wasn't famous, and he didn't own a fancy car or house, but he could get a squirrel to eat out of his hand and to him that was far more important.

Dementia robbed me of my father and robbed him of his life. I know that when I take Dad into dinner tonight, he won't even remember I was there ten minutes after I leave. But in this moment, he knows I'm here and he knows he loves squirrels. So we feed the squirrels. Every Wednesday.

~Rhonda Penders

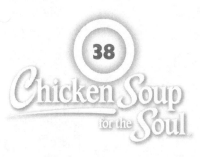

My Mother's Eyes

The eyes are the window to your soul.
~William Shakespeare

As I head into the nursing home driveway I see the first "Visitor" parking space is open and I pull in. You'd think I'd have a "Reserved" spot after coming here almost every day for the past five years. I walk up, hit the button and go through the door like I've done so many times before. It doesn't get any easier, day after day, year after year.

I see her sitting in her wheelchair at the end of the hall. I kneel down in front of Mom and tell her hello and how much I love her. I look at the familiar crooked smile on her face and I pause at her eyes. She is in her eighteenth year of Alzheimer's disease and is now confined to a wheelchair. When I look at her I don't see how old she has gotten. I don't notice the two missing front teeth she has grinded out due to the dementia. I don't notice how thin her hair has become. I just see my mom.

I see in her eyes the same pride she had for me decades ago as she sat on the bleachers cheering me on though my sporting events. She always told me you have to learn to lose before you can be a good winner. I see the love she felt as she rolled my hair every Saturday night in those pink sponge curlers for Sunday Mass. I see the laughter in her eyes as she pushed me into the lake to get her cane pole that broke in half while we were fishing. And I see the worried look in her eyes from those nights I snuck into the house after missing curfew.

I wonder what she sees now. As I set up her tray to feed her supper, I wonder if she sees me putting pepper on her food because before Alzheimer's she loved pepper. I wonder if she notices I wash her face and hands before the meal because before Alzheimer's she was always such a tidy lady. Does she see how patient I am as she takes more time to eat than all the other residents? Is that because she always waited to make sure my siblings and I had enough food before she took seconds?

I wonder if she sees me brush her hair and try to style what little is left. Before Alzheimer's she had her hair styled every Friday. I wonder if she sees that I straighten her closet. And I wonder if she sees that I remove all the tags in her gowns because after two or three washings at the nursing home the tags get stiff and scratchy. And if she sees I take her clothes home every couple of weeks and soak them in fabric softener. I wonder if she sees I iron her name patches on the top of her socks so the patches don't tickle her feet.

I wonder if she sees me struggle with the parent-child role reversal as I am forced to make decisions about her health and wellbeing on her behalf. And if I make a mistake with her care, does she forgive me? Does she notice that before I leave the nursing home each night I kiss her, tell her how much I love her, and that God loves her, too?

Because before Alzheimer's became her life that is what she did for me every night as she tucked me into bed.

I wonder—but only for a moment. Because I am sure she does. I can see it in my mother's eyes.

~Theresa Hettinger

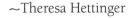

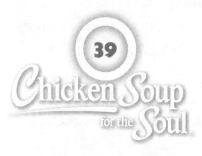

39

Rewind

A daughter is a gift of love.
~Author Unknown

When I was young, a long time ago
You walked with me nice and slow
You held my hand to keep me safe
And made your steps small to suit my pace

Now it's my turn to do that for you
I hold your hand, it's the least I can do
I walk with you up and down the hall
To keep you from stumbling and taking a fall

You squeeze my hand and smile at me
I squeeze yours back just as gently
You don't know my name, but that's okay
Little by little your memory's slipping away

We're on a journey we didn't choose
I realize each day how much we have to lose
You're slowly traveling back in time
I'm watching your life slowly rewind

Your memories are fading, but I'm still here
Though I know shortly, too, I'll disappear

I'll be erased, no matter how tight I hang on
Your grip will grow weak, but I'll remain strong

I'll hold your hand, I'll keep you safe
I'll keep my steps small to suit your pace
No matter what happens we'll walk side by side
We'll travel together this long goodbye.

~Kala Cota

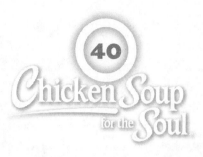

40

A Good Conversation

The most important thing in communication is to hear what isn't being said.
~Peter F. Drucker

ords were the first thing to go. Mom covered it up well, though. As I visited one Saturday, she dragged me into her bedroom and opened the closet door. Smiling, she showed me an outfit she had recently purchased: black slacks and a matching black and red top.

"We went shopping yesterday at… you know, that store where we like to shop." The name of the store had vanished, and I didn't know which store she meant, but it didn't matter. Even without the name, Mom managed to communicate.

After many years with vascular dementia, she spoke less and less. As she lost more and more words, communication became difficult. My once outgoing and social mother struggled to converse. "Baby… heart… store… pretty…" Words that once were strung together to communicate her thoughts now bounced around like a broken strand of pearls.

One day at a family dinner I had a revelation that helped me communicate with Mom. The dinner table at Mom and Dad's house was crowded with children and grandchildren. As dishes were passed and silverware clinked, conversation flowed and laughter erupted. Stories were shared and family members poked good-natured fun at one another.

That's when I noticed. I looked at Mom, who couldn't join in the conversation. Her mouth was set in a stern line and her eyes flashed. She didn't say a word, but I knew she was angry.

When it dawned on me why, I was ashamed. Even though Mom no longer had the ability to carry on a conversation, she still wanted to be included. Because she wasn't talking, we had ignored her. During that entire meal, I hadn't made eye contact with her, nor had anyone else at the table. We had treated her as if she didn't exist.

I couldn't do anything to help Mom regain her ability to use words, but I could include her and communicate with her. I looked into her baby blue eyes, smiled, and nodded my head. Immediately the stern mouth turned upward into a smile. Together, we learned to communicate. She uttered a string of words, "See... car... Mom... walk... boy..." and I responded as if I knew what she was saying.

For a year or two after that, Mom and I had some wonderful conversations. Making eye contact, I smiled at her. I nodded, as if I understood her disjointed words. Gesturing with my hands, I answered her, "Oh, that's funny," and laughed out loud. "Tell me more," I said, and listened attentively to random words that made no sense.

Yes, Mom had lost the ability to convey meaning with her words. But I learned an important truth: We didn't need coherent sentences to communicate, because the language of love doesn't need words.

~Nancy Hamilton Sturm

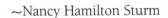

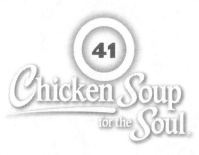

41

In Your Winter Kitchen

To live in hearts we leave behind is not to die.
~Thomas Campbell

Because of you,
and the recipe you once wrote for me
in your elegant hand,
I bought bittersweet chocolate in the store today,
hazelnut spread, and heavy cream.
In the afternoon we will bake mousse cake, warm
your house against the blowing cold and early-dark
of winter. Light from your kitchen windows will spill out
on bony trees, on tight-furled leaves
of rhododendron, and you will ask me who
I am, and I will think of
yet more things I didn't know to ask you
when I could have,
and I will believe we can inhale the memories
drifting in the chocolate air.

~Jennifer L. Freed

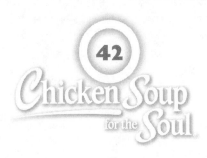

The Hand that Feeds

All the art of living lies in a fine mingling of letting go and holding on.
~Havelock Ellis

t is Friday afternoon and traffic on Golf Road is starting to build. I am immune to it as I travel west, against the flow. I pass the shopping mall, horse barn, museum, and construction zones. My thoughts are on my dad as I near the nursing home. I greet Carol at the desk, check Dad's mail, and make my way to The Neighborhood, where the residents who have Alzheimer's and dementia live. I press the code and enter the secure unit.

This afternoon, the other residents are out in the living room watching Animal Planet. I wave to Alfred, and he smiles. I tell Ellie that her necklace is beautiful and she hugs me. I take Judy's hand, and for a moment she stops shaking.

I knock on Dad's door, and enter. It's 5:30 p.m., and he has been up from his afternoon nap for about an hour. Now, he's consumed with pain. Jeff, his private duty caregiver, tells me that Dad was complaining about his ankles so they are propped up on the footstool. I thank Jeff and hand him his weekly check—ever since Dad's strokes, Jeff has been instrumental in nursing Dad back to life. I check the diaper supply and stock the fridge with Ensure. Dad is leaning back in his wheelchair, eyes closed, mouth open. I hear a moan, and I walk over, sit on the bed and take his hand.

Music is one of my best ways to communicate with him so I start singing to him about Daisy and the bicycle built for two. My pitch and tone are way off, but I don't care. It's one of our favorite songs, and after a minute his eyes open. I ask him if he's ever ridden a bicycle built for two. He says no, and I remind him how he used to put our dog Rusty in the grocery basket of his old bike and give him rides around Evanston. Finally, I get a smile. Then the moaning starts again.

I ask where it hurts: this time, it's his shoulders. Jeff says he's already had his pain medicine and we're waiting for it to kick in. I ask Jeff if the hospice volunteer came today. He says yes; Dad says no. I believe Jeff. I put on some music. Ellington. We've changed the words a bit.

In our version, it's "If you want to get from Sugar Hill to Harlem, you better take the A train." We sit. His hands are soft. Softer than mine. His arms are splotched with purple and red marks. I take note of a few new bruises and cuts.

It's dinnertime, and lately Dad has been taking his meals in his room. Jeff brings in some soup. Tomato barley. I stir it, taste it, and scald my tongue. After a few minutes it's ready and I ask Dad to open his mouth. He does, takes a bite of soup and makes a horrible face but it stays mostly in his mouth. He chews for almost a minute and I wonder how that's possible. I don't see him swallow, but the chewing stops. I try with another spoonful, and another. Four more bites and he's had enough. The bib is covered with spills. I wipe his mouth and nose. I haven't seen him eat this much in months. Jeff brings in his plate.

Chicken and mashed potatoes. I know Jeff usually ends up feeding him Ensure, yogurt, and dessert—that seems to be all Dad will take these days. But I'm here, so we try for solid food and whole nutrition. And he eats. It surprises even me, but his eyes are closed and he's reluctantly accepting every bite I bring to his mouth. Chew, chew, drool, chew, spit, moan, chew, swallow.

With each bite I feed him, I am reminded of what his doctors and the hospice team keep saying—as long as he has nutrition and is able to take food, he could survive for quite some time. And I think of the pain he is in. And I think of the loneliness in his eyes when I'm not there. And I wonder if what I'm doing is helping or hurting. He is chewing, swallowing, digesting. He is surviving. But is that what he wants? Is it worth it?

Jeff sees that his plate is almost empty and remarks again how special our connection is. "He doesn't eat like that for me," he says. And I can't smile, because my stomach is churning.

I have to leave. Suddenly I don't feel safe here. I clean off his mouth, give him a kiss, tell him I love him. He smiles, unable to say it back but I know he's thinking it. I type the code and bolt out the door. Back in the car I punch the stations—NPR, XRT, there has to be something to clear my mind, because I can't handle silence right now.

I find Wilco and settle in for the twenty-minute drive home. I stop at Mom's long enough to guzzle a glass of wine and pick up the laundry I did earlier in the day. Then I'm on my way, alone with my thoughts. Fighting with myself over the need to hold on and the need to let go.

~Carrie Jackson

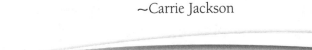

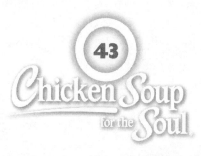

Always a Mother

Mother is a verb, not a noun.
~Proverb

had just heard two of the most dreaded words in the English language. "It's cancer." My husband gripped my hand, as I struggled not to dissolve into tears. I want my mother, my inner child wailed. I craved the reassurance, the support that only a mother could give.

But she was the one person I couldn't turn to. Her home was hundreds of miles away, and she lived in the fog of Alzheimer's.

For more than five years the dementia had stalked her, ripping away memory and severing logic, leaving confusion and fear in its wake. During those years, she'd become the child. I mothered her through bouts of panic, when she couldn't remember where her home was. I comforted her when she cried as she relived her own mother's death. I calmed her when dementia-induced fear erupted in a temper tantrum. I metaphorically tucked her into bed each night, sending her kisses over the phone line while my own heart fractured.

Now, when dementia gnawed on her mind and cancer ate away at my body, numb hopelessness enveloped me. I didn't dare let the word cancer slip into the daily conversations with my mother.

Yet she knew things weren't right, and the protective wall I'd built around her began to crumble. At first it was a tiny chink, brought about by her insistence that something was wrong with me. The chink cracked and widened until the wall crashed down. She demanded I tell her my secrets. I stopped holding back and shared the news of my impending surgery—still careful not to use the "C" word, but admitting my other fears.

She asked if I'd have a scar.

Yes, I would.

"Well," she said, "I think a diamond necklace should cover it nicely."

I smiled.

Together with my stepfather, she made the 500-mile trek to my house to "help" me through the treatments. On the eve of my surgery, family surrounded me.

At the hospital, as the team prepared to wheel me away, my mother pushed past my husband to grab my hand. "I love you," she whispered fiercely, her eyes blazing as she bent close and kissed my cheek. In that moment, the tears I'd held at bay for months broke free and the fear loosened its grip.

By some miracle, my mother had thrown off the dementia, fighting her way through the fog to be at my side. She'd come to me when I needed her most. Her spirit was stronger than the disease.

The moment of grace lasted through the hours of surgery and beyond. During the night, my husband sat at my bedside, while my mother and stepfather managed alone in my house, without the benefit of their routine. They stayed with us through the days of recovery until I was home and safe.

Then, the fog descended again. Dementia locked my mother away and I returned to parenting her. But with a difference.

She'd taught me something. This, her last and best lesson, was that the mind might fail. The body may deteriorate. But the spirit will remain strong.

As she slipped further away from us in mind and body, I began to watch for glimpses of that indomitable spirit. Sometimes, it tiptoed in with flashes of humor. Once, while visiting, I lost my train of thought. "I'm sorry, sweetheart," she said as she smiled and patted my hand. "I didn't know it was contagious."

At other times it stomped in with a stubborn declaration. "You're not the boss of me!" my mother shouted when I encouraged her to take a hated medicine.

But mostly, it appeared in her constant determination to live life on her terms. She fought to stay with her family, surrendering to death only on her terms, and in her time. She left surrounded by her children, husband, and friends—that spirit still intact.

Even today, her spirit whispers to me that nothing—neither death nor dementia—can stand in the way of love.

~Kelle Z. Riley

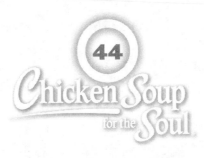

Love Is the Answer

Be completely humble and gentle;
Be patient, bearing with one another in love.
~Ephesians 4:2

My mother-in-law, whom I called Grandma for twenty-five years, was a true Southern mom. Cooking was a gift she gave her family daily. The meals were routine—sausage gravy with biscuits, fried chicken, salmon patties, and chicken-fried steak. If you wanted fried potatoes or any of the above at midnight, she would make them with a smile on her face. The moment her feet hit the floor, the bacon and eggs hit the pan. This was her routine every morning, despite the fact that she lived alone for forty years. Widowed at age forty-five, she chose never to date again. There was only one love in her life—her husband of twenty-four years and the father of her two sons.

Unfortunately, Alzheimer's disease stole Grandma's independence. When she was no longer able to live alone, my husband and I agreed to ask her to stay with us. We made this decision with some misgivings, as we realized our own freedom would be limited. But Grandma's freedom had been taken from her forever by Alzheimer's.

When Grandma came to live with us, my husband and I decided to keep her bacon and egg routine going. On the first morning, my feet hit the floor early and into the kitchen I went. The bacon had just started to sizzle, the wonderful aroma filling the air, when I heard a voice from behind. "Good morning, Nancy, I'm here!"

Looking up, my eyes met Grandma's. And looking back at me were eyes as black as black could be. She had gone to bed with white, sparse eyebrows, and now she had eyebrows like Groucho Marx. Apparently she had done her make-up with a hidden Marks-A-Lot marker rather than Maybelline, to create lasting color around her eyes.

Of course, I didn't say a word about it. Reassurance and security are things my mother-in-law needs daily. Jingle bells, secured to her walker, alert us to her wanderings. Some nights we awaken to every light on in the house as she jingles her way into our bedroom. Peering in, she sweetly asks, "Are you there?"

We gently reassure her and she returns to bed. Sometimes a kiss and tucking-in is all she needs. Other nights my husband must awaken fully and talk with her to calm her.

Grandma takes full responsibility for her dog, Happy. We no longer count the number of times we answer her question, "Where's Happy? Happy can't get out, can he?" One night I heard her feeding Happy at 3 a.m. The next morning, I found birdseed in his dish. She has lived with us almost two years now, yet often looks at us quizzically and says, "I had a nice time, but Happy and I need to get home."

There are times I become frustrated—when her clothes are dirty, or her Depends need changing, yet she remains unaware. It's then my eyes go to the photographs on her bedroom wall and my impatience softens. I see a beautiful young wife, vacationing with her husband in Colorado, wearing a starched blouse and a skirt, with hose and pumps. That lady is still in there. On good days we still see her.

Grandma occupies her time doing word searches, looking after Happy, watching movies with me or Rangers baseball with her son. On good days she cannot get enough to eat and whatever I cook is met with, "This is my favorite." We are blessed, as she is easy to please and remains in good spirits (most of the time). After all, we all have our moments, don't we?

Well-meaning friends and family members are the first to ask about our new roles as caregivers. We tell them we have learned a lot over the past two years. We have put into practice the words of wisdom I learned as a nurse and a flight attendant: "Put on your own oxygen mask before assisting others."

As caregivers, we take time out to pursue what we enjoy. We visit with family and find sitters to stay with Grandma. We enjoy gardening, reading, writing, walking our dog, Zoey, or simply going out for coffee. We commit to taking care of ourselves.

It has been a challenge to grasp Grandma's hand and walk confidently with her through these last pages of her life. We keep our eyes open to see the blessings she brings into our days and the wisdom she shares along the way. After all, there are still things she can teach us… like who knew a Marks-A-Lot would give far more lasting color than Maybelline?

As each day closes, Grandma sits on her bed, reading and rereading cards sent by her sons, granddaughters, grandsons, and daughters-in-law. Looking up as I say goodnight, she whispers, "Remember, love is the answer."

~Nancy King Barnes

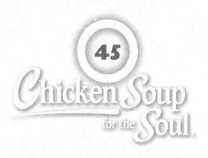

Learning Acceptance

*You can clutch the past so tightly to your chest
that it leaves your arms too full to embrace the present.*
~Jan Glidewell

Mom was everything to me: best friend, confidante, trusted advisor, and my biggest cheerleader. Hearing her say she was proud of the mother I had become to my own daughter was tantamount to winning the most prestigious honor on earth.

Despite the closeness we shared, I'm sure I took her and our relationship for granted more often than I'd like to admit. It's what we do. We get wrapped up in our busy lives, succumb to everyday stresses, and operate as though our loved ones will always be there. And then, something like Alzheimer's comes along and turns our world upside down.

Of course I knew my mother wouldn't live forever, but things unfolded in a way I never imagined. We were supposed to have another twenty years to travel, shop, and bake together. We think of Alzheimer's as a disease of the elderly, but Mom was barely sixty-seven. I didn't understand what was happening and there was such a sense of denial, frustration, and anger.

At first, it was almost like being returned to the turmoil of my teen years. My initial reaction was that she had somehow caused this by not staying active enough when she retired. I made a calendar for her and filled each week with activities—my way of encouraging her to "keep moving." Most of it was ignored. Now I look back and wonder if she was failing much sooner than we realized and the withdrawal was a function of the disease rather than vice versa.

There's no question that our relationship suffered until I finally reached a point of acceptance. I had to stop expecting her to "try harder" and "do more." I had to accept that she couldn't help what was happening to her, and most of all I had to adjust to the fact that she was becoming the child, and I, the parent. In hindsight, I wish I could have done all of those things sooner than I did—so much time was wasted.

Ultimately, however, our connection was strengthened exponentially, and I felt closer to her than ever before. It's a testament to the fact that even immense loss and heartbreak can bring blessings.

Although she lost her speech very early on, we managed to communicate until the end, whether through an affectionate look, a shared smile, or a gentle touch. And every once in a while, in a gift of all gifts, she would manage to say, "I love you."

Alzheimer's teaches us the fundamental meaning of compassion, acceptance, and unconditional love. It shows us that even the most ordinary experiences can be extraordinary, and although the pain of losing someone to this disease is indescribable, it reminds us that not a single moment should be taken for granted.

Almost a year after her passing, I treasure the simple things more than ever. In a world of instant gratification, material belongings, and confused priorities, we tend to forget that tomorrow is not promised. I still have my moments, but clear perspective now rises closer to the surface than ever before.

Thank you, Mom, for continuing to be my teacher and constant source of strength and inspiration—today and always.

~Ann Napoletan

You will face unique challenges when it comes to family, work, finances and future care. But you have the power to make a new plan and determine how you chose to live your best life with the disease.

"If You Have Younger-Onset Alzheimer's Disease"
www.alz.org/youngeronest

Chapter 6

Living with Alzheimer's

& Other Dementias

Younger-Onset Alzheimer's

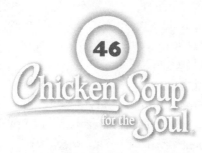

The Hardest Day

*You have to leave the city of your comfort and go into
the wilderness of your intuition. What you'll discover will be wonderful.
What you'll discover is yourself.*

~Alan Alda

On a spring morning in April 2001, I sat in the doctor's
reception room anxiously waiting for her to emerge
with my husband after two intense days of testing. She
asked me to speak to her privately in her office and said,
"Mrs. Henley, I am so sorry to have to tell you, but your husband has
Alzheimer's disease." Then she brought Mike in and went over her
findings with him as well. The fear I'd had for months was true, but
how could this happen? Mike was only thirty-six years old.

Back in the car, in tears, I discussed our situation with Mike.
"How are the kids going to handle this?" he asked. Courtney and
Brandon were only nine and seven years old, respectively. Most adults
don't understand this disease. How were we to expect our children
would?

"It's okay to put me in a nursing home," was Mike's second comment. Then he added, "I want you to remarry."

Part of me felt like I was living in an alternate universe, not
knowing what to say or do. How were the kids going to handle this?
Without him working, would I lose the house? We struggled for years
on two salaries; how could I survive on one?

Alzheimer's disease had always been a fear lurking in the back of my mind since Mike's mom had been diagnosed in 1985 at age forty-five. Her diagnosis came as a shock to the family, because no one had had it before her.

We didn't know at the time that she had familial Alzheimer's and passed to each of her children a fifty percent chance of inheriting the gene. When Mike said I had his permission to put him in a nursing home, it was based on his own mother's struggle, which he dealt with when he was nineteen. His mom had spent the seven years after diagnosis in a nursing home and passed away at age fifty-two.

I thought this was the absolute hardest day of our lives. So many questions and fears ran through my mind and the path ahead looked bleak. Many friends and family disappeared from our lives, but those who stuck around were nothing short of angelic. Their love, support, and help were simply miraculous.

At the end of the day, it was my faith in God and all he had planned for me that kept me going. I am proud to say that my children and I cared for Mike at home for the eleven years he struggled through this disease. It was definitely not easy, but it's something I would never change. My children were active co-caregivers, and I couldn't be more proud of them. Mike passed away at home on February 28, 2012, at age forty-seven.

The Hardest Day

I thought the day he received the diagnosis would be the hardest.
Then I realized it would be the day we had to tell our children.
Little did I know that this disease would bring many more "hardest"
    days.

I'm still not sure on whom it was harder—
my handsome, lovable, generous thirty-six-year-old husband,
The man who adored his son and daughter more than life itself,
knowing he would never see them grow up to be the most amazing
    adults.
The man who had already lost his mom to the disease,

yet who accepted his fate with grace.
My hero, who lost his voice way too soon
who endured countless hospitalizations from an illness that ravaged
his body and mind.

Or was it harder on me —
His wife of thirteen years and his full-time caregiver,
As I watched my soul mate engulfed in a disease that showed no
mercy?
My heart broke with each forgotten thought, each unfinished
sentence,
and when his frustration would grow into an act of agitation.
I cried each night as I held his hand while he slept beside me,
wondering if he knew it was me who was with him.
I mourned my husband each and every day
I mourned all we had hoped we would have and all that Alzheimer's
disease took from us.

Sadder than all of this —
I feel it was hardest on our children.
Imagine being seven and nine years old and being told your dad was
going to forget you,
even though he loved you very much.
Imagine the fear of seeing your kind-hearted, fun-loving dad
become so agitated that he put his fist through a wall.
Imagine what it was like to feed your father
when you were only thirteen and he was forty.
Picture being a child and having the one person you loved and looked
up to most in the world
ripped away from you, day by day, to a disease too horrific to
imagine.

There are too many hardest days when dealing with Alzheimer's
disease.
The day they forget who you are

The day their voice goes silent
The day they can no longer walk
The day they become incontinent
The day they can't feed themselves
The day the bedsores start
The day they start to choke

And the day they lose the battle.

Rest peacefully Mike—we love you and will never forget you.
Our hero.

~Karen M. Henley

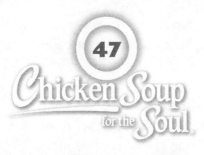

The Promises We Make

What a happy and holy fashion it is that those who love one another
should rest on the same pillow.
~Nathaniel Hawthorne

I remember the moment my world changed. I was working a long day in the city, and my wife delighted me with the promise of my favorite dinner. Tonight, she said, we would have roasted red peppers, fresh mozzarella, and basil, with some olive oil and balsamic vinegar, and a loaf of fresh Italian bread from the bakery.

I walked in the door that evening, anticipating our delicious meal, and to my surprise, the table only held two place settings and a loaf of bread. Nothing else. And no indication from my wife that anything was amiss. That moment confirmed what I had suspected for a while. I wanted to cry, wrap my arms around my wife, and beg her to please, please, not disappear on me. But there was no getting around it. My wife had younger-onset Alzheimer's.

That was three years ago, when she was only fifty-one. Now at fifty-four, she continues her long, slow descent into a place where my will to bring her back has no effect.

My nickname for Linda is Radio Bean, a play on Radiant Being. I have never known another person to be so joyful, optimistic, and radiant. As time has passed, I have witnessed the struggle inside her between that joyful woman and the mysterious dark force that's descending, smothering her personality. The image it creates for me is of my beautiful wife drowning, reaching out with her hand to me, looking intensely into my eyes for me to save her. But I can't. Therein lies the heartbreak. But what I have discovered is that she could save me, completing the selfless promise of love she always reserved for me.

Our life these days is all about re-membering. Not remembering events, but rather a coming together of the most essential, sacred aspects of ourselves in a way that gives meaning and relevance to our struggle. Our challenge with this illness is to pave a way to something of value that underscores the strength of our love for each other.

While she forgets, I learn to re-member. In a way I am re-membering for both of us; for as she loses her identity, she feebly latches onto mine. She turns to me to not only take care of her worldly needs, but also to validate her state. If I am happy, she is happier. If I am peaceful, she is more internally relaxed.

So why not use this emotional tether to lead us both into a deeper state of grace? Why not take her hand, and stumble together toward the light? And stumble we do. Because as any caregiver who has gone through this knows, it is a road fraught with frustration, impatience, sadness, and resentment.

The one question that never seems to have an answer is, why? Why her? Why me? Strength then, must come in searching for grace in the absence of understanding. I might never know why. But what I do know is that none of what she does, doesn't do, says, or doesn't say is her fault. I also know that I made her a promise to love and cherish her in sickness and in health. And that promise doesn't mean we simply stick it out. It underscores our assurance to continue to march into the light and rail against the unrelenting forces that seek to undermine our resolve.

On her worst days I see much less of her in her eyes. She responds to me less, disappearing more. I find myself praying that she is retreating to a place that is peaceful for her.

When she sleeps, I gently kiss her on the lips and forehead and quietly plead with her to come back to me. I wish she could hitch a ride on a passing miracle in her dreams and ride it home to me where I will be waiting with kisses and gifts and adventures.

At the same time, I lay my head down and remember that our deal with life is for all of it, not just the warm and fuzzy stuff. So I contemplate patience, and I reflect on love, and I discover that while my life may look different than anything I could have imagined years ago, I am still blessed. I am still grateful to have a wife who has been the great love of my life. Who is as beautiful in illness as she is in health, because I know her and I know that somewhere in there, she remains.

Alzheimer's is a dreadful disease. It takes away what is so precious. It derails lives and steals dreams. But it is also an opportunity to discover the truest meaning of love, of patience, and ultimately to find our best selves. I know how easy it was to recite vows on our wedding day. I now know how difficult it is to see those vows put to the test. But now at least I know what a vow means. Now at least I know what a life means. And now, at least, I know what love means.

Three years into it, my Radio Bean is still with me. We are still us. There is certainly enough awareness that we can still share so much, and we do—long drives in the country, movies, dinner with great, compassionate friends. We love to go hiking. We walk down the street holding hands. But now, we are holding much more than hands. We are holding on to each other and the promise we made.

Alzheimer's takes away so much. And in some strange way, it gives as well—as long as we stay open to grace and are willing to appreciate that there are some answers we might never have.

~Dr. David Davis

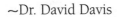

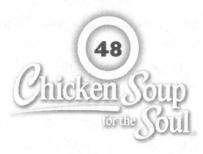

Finding Dad

Don't wait to make your son a great man — make him a great boy.
~Author Unknown

I was twelve and Dad had been sick for a few years. Now he looked old, more bent over. His face was lined and his black hair was slowly starting to gray, but it was mostly his eyes; those big friendly deep brown eyes were so sad-looking, without the sparkle they used to have.

And when he went for a walk he had trouble remembering how to get home.

Sometimes Mom would call us in from playing to go look for him and bring him back. My younger brother Bruce and I would split up and walk through the neighborhood trying to act as if we weren't really out tracking our father.

One particular time stands out. It was a chilly autumn day, and I had my jacket zipped up against the cold. I shuffled along the sidewalk, vaguely avoiding each concrete crack. The idea that they were expansion joints there to save the walkway didn't lessen their mystic significance from those "break your mother's back" rhymes. I was wary of the possibilities — my life was damaged enough already.

With luck, Dad wouldn't be too far and I could get back to my games or continue building forts before the weekend ran out. I trailed along our street, heading in the direction I thought I would most likely find him. I always sent Bruce the other way; maybe then he wouldn't have to deal with Dad. He was only seven, but he knew not to go too far and compound the problem of people being lost.

Our life had two realities: before Dad got sick, and after.

Before, life felt positive, Mom was happy; things were generally good. Afterward, sadness pervaded, even in the good times. Dad was slowly getting worse, a constant reminder of how bad it was—for him, for us, and for the future.

In a lot of ways, we took it in stride. I learned not to feel overwhelmed by responsibilities I couldn't handle; my brother learned to stay empowered by feeling angry at life's unfairness.

As the older brother I was lucky enough to have quite a few fuzzy but good memories of Dad. I knew he loved us enough to have built us a sandbox, then built a sunroof over it and decorated it with pictures of horses and Native Americans—the first time I figured out my father could draw that well. He taught me the rudiments of perspective with a dot trick for drawing cubes, and how to play "The Bear Went Over the Mountain" on the harmonica. My brother, five years younger, couldn't remember much of the time before the disease.

On this particular Saturday search there was no one out on our street, and I found him in ten minutes, striding along in his slippers and sweater. Luckily, he was still short of the busy main street. By now he was probably cold. I walked up to him and touched his arm and he sort of recognized me, but was muttering in confusion. It was hard to know what he was thinking or where he might have thought he was going.

"Come on, Dad," I said quietly. "Let's go home."

I was hoping he would comply easily and not attract attention, but he pulled his arm away, muttering unhappily. I took a breath and touched his arm again. This time he started moving slowly with me back toward our house.

He still towered over me then, but I was never afraid of him. There was no threat of violence in him toward us. He could be immovable, but he would never lash out.

I began to relax as we made our way back up the street, but then

Dad stopped. I could only watch and look around frantically as Dad unzipped and began to pee right there on the sidewalk in front of someone's house.

"Dad, you can't do that," I wailed, but I knew it was way too late. The embarrassment was excruciating, and I'm sure I felt a fleeting impulse to run, but I couldn't do that, either. There was nothing to do but stand with him until he finished and I could get him moving again.

We got home without further incident. But I could never relax after that—you never knew when something like that might happen again.

Dad tried hard throughout his illness. Over and over he would repeat the litany of our names, "Paul and Bruce and Margaret." He must have made a conscious decision to nail at least these few crucial facts as he felt so many others fade. It hurts me now to imagine how frightening that must have been for him. But his determination prevailed and he had those words until he died.

We knew he loved us right to the end.

~Paul Hyckie

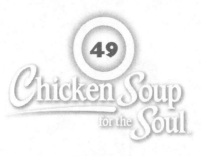

Life on 24th Street

Although it's difficult today to see beyond the sorrow,
May looking back in memory help comfort you tomorrow.
~Author Unknown

I was going through an old box the other day when I ran across an envelope full of coupons. My mother had written notes on the back of the envelope.

"Call piano movers," one said. Another described life on our old street: "The sound of the wind in winter as it gusts and swishes through the enormously tall fir tree, with an echo as the garage door occasionally sucks air under it. The utter peace as I pull into our vast secluded driveway—the promise of privacy; of space to walk within the house and in the gracious calm yard."

Yet another, now distinct note: "Something urges me to move, it's time, but I don't quite understand why, but I feel like I need to follow the urge."

"Goodbye Dear Home. 11-29-93"

Two months later my mom moved out of our family home and began a new life she was unsure about.

My mom had turned forty-nine six days before 11-29-93. Did she know something was happening to her? That something was awry? She described the strange changes in herself as an urge. Was it an urge for a new beginning? Or was it an urge for someone or something to recreate the calm she had known before something started to go awry inside her brain?

Not long after that move, my mom started doing odd things—scribbling notes on Post-its, forgetting appointments, having trouble balancing the checkbook and paying bills on time, and making mistakes at the office.

Now, ten years later, when I run into people from the old neighborhood they ask how my mom is doing. They think I will say she fell in love again after losing my beloved father—she at forty-one, he at forty-five. They think I will say something about how she spends her time playing tennis like she did in the old days, or enjoying time with her grandchildren.

But my response only deepens their sadness for my mom. That she no longer recognizes her children or her brothers and sisters. That she never knew all her grandchildren, or her daughter-in-law. I say that we are happy for the great care she gets in her adult family home.

This past Tuesday my mom went into the hospital after another seizure. We are discovering the wear and tear that Alzheimer's has inflicted on her once muscular body, and she is experiencing the start of kidney and liver failure.

This past Thursday I prayed to God. I asked him to take care of my mother. To make the pain stop. She does not deserve this. She is the woman who cared for a two-year-old and newborn twins at the same time. The woman who raised three teenagers as a widow. The woman who won round-robin tournaments, chaired the board of a country club, and ran a business when the boss had to leave town. She is the woman who appreciated what was given to her in life, including the gracious calm moments of peace.

She deserves this peace.

My mother, just shy of fifty-nine years old, finally gave in to the assurances of God and her children that everything would be okay. Not a day goes by when I don't think of her, and miss her terribly. And I am comforted knowing she found her calm and peaceful place once again.

~Susie Van Den Ameele

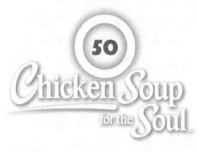

Bring Him to Me

In union there is strength.

~Aesop

My husband John was fifty-four when he was diagnosed with younger-onset Alzheimer's disease. John was young, gifted, and talented. A loving husband, dad, brother, and friend.

Within a year he had to retire from the industry where we had met thirty-three years before. We were shocked. What would life be like?

When first diagnosed, John was still able to drive, so he would sometimes go to the driving range or come by the office so we could go to lunch. He also spent his days working around the house and taking care of the yard.

Then he began spending time with an acquaintance of ours who had recently lost his wife. Ray was no longer able to drive, so John started out taking him out once a week for breakfast, which soon turned into three days a week for breakfast and lunch. A beautiful new friendship had begun.

Then the time came when our doctor told John he could no longer drive. Although John seemed to take the news pretty well, my new concern was what would he do all day at home alone? He was so used to being around others.

On the way home from the doctor's office we stopped by Ray's house and the three of us went to dinner. When John stepped away from the table, I told Ray the news. I explained that John would no longer be able to come by and that my only option would be to take John to an adult day center during the days while I was at work. That's when our dear friend said these four sweet words: "Bring him to me."

Starting the next day, I began taking John to Ray's house, and the two of them would spend their days together. Other friends and family members would stop by several times a week and take them both to breakfast or lunch. Some days, I would stop on the way home from work and pick up dinner for the three of us, only to arrive and hear the sweet sound of the two of them singing along while watching the Gaithers performing on television.

They spent lots of time together enjoying each other's company and reflecting on days of their past. But once John started to wander, a common behavior of Alzheimer's disease, I had to start taking him to an adult day center. We would still visit Ray or take him dinner and the three of us would cry when Ray would tell John how much he loved and missed him.

John continues to attend the adult day center; however, our sweet friend Ray passed away this past March at age ninety. His words, "Bring him to me," will remain with me always.

~Susan Young

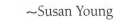

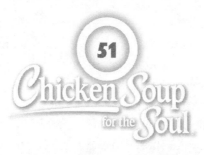

Runaway Words

Language is the blood of the soul into which thoughts run
and out of which they grow.
~Oliver Wendell Holmes

y husband Jack was a man of few words, which is a funny thing to say about someone who adored them. Quiet and introspective, he loved everything about words—quirky spellings, pronunciation and, of course, their meanings and origins. The man was not a bookworm but a book python, devouring the printed word in all forms, digesting every vocabulary word that came his way. He read two newspapers every day, did *The New York Times* crossword puzzles, and subscribed to countless magazines, including *The New Yorker*, *Harper's*, *The Atlantic*, and *The Smithsonian*.

Jack was also a bit of a word snob, and liked to throw them around from time to time in our blue-collar city. He often introduced me to people by saying, "Rose is a peach and that's a conundrum!"

Later, when our daughter came along, he referred to us both as his "Peachy girls!" Once, we got into a crowded elevator in a city hospital. An uncomfortable silence had fallen over the shoulder-to-shoulder group, when Jack announced loudly, "I did not like that doctor. He was too effusive!"

From the back of the crowd, a man said, "What a great word!" They laughed together and shared a hearty handshake as though they were members of some secret lexical brotherhood.

Jack read with a little notepad by his side and wrote down words as he went along. Sometimes they were words he didn't know, but mostly they were words that caught his fancy and he wanted to research later. I recently found a slip of paper, three inches by three inches, with sixty-two words on the front and back, written in his neat printing. Such words as cupidity, threnody, miasma, and pullulating fill this scrap, most crossed through to indicate completed homework. This reading was done before online dictionaries: his battered three-inch-thick *Living Webster Encyclopedic Dictionary* was his constant reading companion.

The man read all eleven volumes of Will and Ariel Durant's *The Story of Civilization* twice, and was attempting it a third time when he was diagnosed with Alzheimer's at age fifty-nine. Jack had to give up his job as an art teacher and together we began a slow journey of losses. But the most tragic for him would be the loss of words. He told me, "The words see me coming and they run away."

At the suggestion of our doctor, Jack and I began to keep journals. Jack's was to help him remember things such as appointments, agreements we made and, most importantly for him, notes about his reading. It frustrated him to read one day and not remember any of it the next. It felt like starting the same book over and over. So many of his journal pages are notes on the topic he read, the dates involved, and the page numbers. I am not sure if he found this helpful.

In Alice Walker's *The Color Purple*, we see the main character Celie grow as a person. Her writing at first is rudimentary and we have to guess at words and meanings. But as time goes on, she gains her voice, learning how to read and write with clarity. Jack's journals, to me, are just the opposite. We see the progression of his long journey, with his spelling and syntax falling to ruin. Examples of his new words include squerills, corderoe, maneuvors, comradite, bran mufee, buryall, and messaric.

After six years at home, our lives became more complicated with a diagnosis of colon cancer. A few months later I had no choice but to place Jack in a nursing home. I would visit him daily after work, watching him become quieter and quieter. Every now and then a window of lucidity would open. I treasured those moments!

Once he told me that seeing me was like going out on a first date, over and over again. Another time he proposed marriage and, when I informed him that we were already married, he said, "Oh, boy! We're going to have fun tonight!"

Gradually he spoke less and less, and then all the words were gone. I can't tell you when I noticed this for good; it just slowly happened. I miss his repartee, his intelligence, his kind and loving words.

After Jack died, I went through his beloved library and sold many of the art and history books to a good friend for his bookstore. I still have his dictionary and the Durant collection. I can't part with them when I know his fingerprints are on every page. I have promised the history set to our son Kevin, and one day the dictionary will go to his peachy girl, Heather. Their dad would be happy to know his treasures have remained in the family. These words are staying right here.

~Rose M. Grant

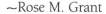

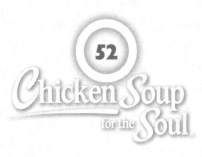

52

The Journey Begins

A teacher affects eternity; he can never tell where his influence stops.
~Henry Brooks Adams

We had known for a little more than a month before we decided to let others in on the burden our family had been carrying. On the last day of school before Thanksgiving break, my husband, at age forty-six, stood before his beloved high school students and told them our horrific secret.

We taught at the same high school, so I was able to be with him as his words first began to spill out during homeroom that morning. "I won't be returning to school after Thanksgiving break, I am taking a medical leave," he began. "I have an incurable brain disease and I am no longer able to continue in this job I love." He never spoke the words "Alzheimer's disease" that day, but he didn't need to. The students knew what he was talking about.

It was painful to stand beside him and watch as my husband of more than twenty years spoke to each of his six social studies classes that day. I could see the chins start to quiver and the tears begin to fall. There was a stunned silence. During that first class, after he told the students, a young lady came up and asked him so meekly, "I know you are my teacher, but for today is it okay if I give you a hug?" And thus began the long line of embraces from students. Some clung to their favorite teacher and sobbed—some of the toughest guys gave some of the most emotional hugs that day.

Makeshift cards from students began to appear as the day went on, and alumni began to show up at his door.

One sweet girl said she wanted to help him and offered to wash his chalkboards. We were out of the classroom when she started and when we returned this is what was written on the chalkboard:

We love you! You are the best teacher EVER! We will miss you sooooooooo much and pray for your family. Love, Your Awesome Students

And so began our journey into the uncharted waters of living with Alzheimer's at age forty-six. The day my sweet husband stood so bravely before his students to explain the onslaught of Alzheimer's will always be a lasting memory to me of his strength, character, and resolve to do what was best for his students and family. I know he wanted to honor God with his honesty and integrity that day—and he did.

~Sandy Morris

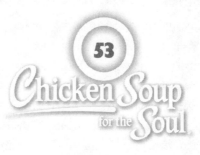

53

On the Road with Alzheimer's

Kindness, like a boomerang, always returns.
~Author Unknown

My husband Bill Bailey was diagnosed with younger-onset Alzheimer's in 2008. Although he was not outwardly suffering from the disease, we both felt disappointment at the changes that were to come.

His career as a research scientist was demanding and he was making more and more mistakes. Reluctantly, he opted for early retirement at age fifty-eight. He found himself facing long days with not enough to do, so he decided to volunteer for the highway department and "adopt" a highway—keeping it clear of litter, and monitoring it with the use of a hard hat, signs, and trash bags.

He was meticulous in his responsibilities, and for more than a year singlehandedly maintained that stretch of road with his long-handled grabber, filling bright orange trash bags to capacity.

The highway department put up a plaque on the part of the highway Bill had adopted, memorializing its adoption by Bill, with the words "Won't You Come Home Bill Bailey," a classic old song.

Then Bill's condition worsened, and he couldn't continue his volunteer work. We were faced with his transition to an assisted living facility. He said the one thing he wished he could take with him was the sign that had his name on it from the highway. In my haze, I considered hatching a plan to unscrew and grab the sign late at night, but my neighbor thought otherwise, suggesting instead we ask for it from the highway department.

To me, that sounded even dumber than my plan. I laughed about my silliness with my co-workers and then put it out of my mind.

Several weeks later a brown paper package arrived on my desk, and inside it was the blue highway sign, "Won't You Come Home Bill Bailey." I broke down, and then my boss told me to take a closer look. The sign had no holes. The highway department had made me a duplicate and told me the original would remain on that stretch of highway in honor of Bill and his dedication. Someone at the highway department had been affected by Alzheimer's disease and helped with this show of kindness.

The sign is now with Bill, in a nursing facility, and its twin is posted on the road along a very well-tended stretch of highway in Bon Air, Virginia.

~Kitty Kennedy

As the disease progresses, your relationship with your spouse or partner will change; however, your connection can still be rich and fulfilling. Spend time together in ways that bring you closer and help you relate.

"Changing roles"
alz.org/care

Living with Alzheimer's & Other Dementias

In Sickness and In Health

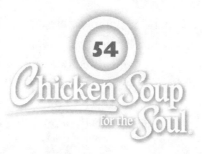

Life Interrupted

*Time, which changes people, does not alter the image
we have retained of them.*

~Marcel Proust

t was the longest one-hour ride Richard and I had ever made, from our home in Richmond, Virginia to the University of Virginia (UVA) medical building. In the past, most of our trips to the university were to attend a meeting, since Richard was on the board of directors. This trip, however, was personal and one we were both dreading.

My husband Richard is well known in the business world. He was chief executive officer of Circuit City stores for twenty years, founder of CarMax, and served as chairman of the board of Crocs, known best for its colorful shoes.

But for me, Richard Sharp has always been the handsome, athletic seventeen-year-old boy I met in high school at age sixteen. As a cheerleader, dating this smart football player was picture perfect! It was literally love at first sight for me. We were married August 17, 1968, and forty-five years later, he is still the love of my life.

No one knows Richard better than I, so when he questioned how to get back home from dinner one night, I knew to be concerned. This day is five years later, in the car on our way to UVA to meet with the doctor for results on neurological tests taken a couple of weeks ago.

While sitting in the doctor's waiting room, I tried to prepare for what I believed to be inevitable news. After being called into his office, the doctor, who Richard knew well following his years of involvement with UVA, looked directly at him and said, "The test shows you are in the early stages of Alzheimer's. I'm sorry."

The doctor then went into a long list of "do's" and "don'ts." I brushed aside the tears that were welling up. It felt more like a verdict than a diagnosis.

"It's important to get your life in order. You will no longer be able to do business where other people's money is involved. You will have to remove yourself from any public boards. You also need to hand over power of attorney involving any personal legal issues."

And then this, the most upsetting question: "How is your driving?" Thankful he had asked the question, I looked at Richard, who replied, "I do all right."

"No Richard, you don't do all right," I said. The look he gave me was one I'd seldom seen in our many years together.

The doctor continued, "Let me ask you a question, Richard. Do you drive with your grandchildren in the car?"

"No," he said.

"So, you won't drive with your own grandchildren in the car but you'll drive on the road where other people's grandchildren may be riding?"

For the first time that afternoon, I saw Richard become visibly emotional. In the years after working hard, his success had afforded him the joy of buying and driving cars that before he could only dream about.

"I have all of my cars. What am I suppose to do with them if I can't drive them?" he asked.

We left the doctor's office and made our way back to the parking lot. Richard handed me the keys to the car and we drove back to Richmond in silence.

When we came into our den, we sat on the sofa, held each other and cried. So many changes we would have to make seemed a daunting task and one for which I personally felt unprepared and ill-equipped.

It has been three years since our visit with the doctor at UVA. We make regular visits to Johns Hopkins and work there with the wonderful doctors and nurses in the neurological department. We know other families are fighting the same battle we fight every day. More than five million people in the United States have Alzheimer's disease, and more than fifteen million are caregivers.

Richard was only sixty-three when he was diagnosed, which is considered younger-onset Alzheimer's disease. His bright mind may be slowly fading, but his energy and optimism remain strong. Our two daughters, their husbands and our four grandchildren have rallied around us with loving support. Some friends give time and expertise, while others provide comic relief, which helps tremendously.

As Richard's primary caregiver, let me shed some light on what I have found to be helpful when looking to the future:

First and foremost, it is my faith that helps keep me going when what I'd really like to do is pull the covers over my head when morning comes. In one of my darkest moments early on, I opened my Bible to read and saw where God promises He will give us "treasures of darkness." I look for these treasures, which are all around us, if we just keep our eyes and hearts open. And because I enjoy photography, I capture the treasures I see.

I've also found it helpful to set a personal goal, every day. A goal that has nothing to do with Alzheimer's disease or the responsibilities that accompany it. It can be time devoted to a hobby, or simply reading a chapter in a favorite book while the person in your care is resting. Or rest yourself.

You may not be able to afford outside help. If this is the case, when friends, family, or others offer their time, receive it as the loving gift it is intended to be without feelings of being a burden. They would not offer if they didn't want to do it. Remember too, your local Alzheimer's Association is available and willing to help whenever possible.

Listen when given advice, but without making any major decision in the moment. Well-meaning friends want to make things better for us by offering ideas. I love my friends and family, but at the end of the day, they all go home and we are left with the reality of our situation. So, "my advice" is to recognize the loving suggestions and then ponder and pray for guidance from God.

Finally, find humor when there's an opportunity for it. Laughter is very healing for everyone, including the person with Alzheimer's. I wish a cure could be that simple.

~Sherry Sharp

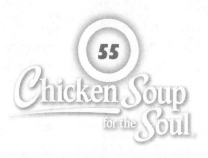

Lessons in the Art of Love

Beauty is not in the face; beauty is a light in the heart.
~Kahlil Gibran

t wasn't until he was in his early eighties that my father taught me about the depths of his love for my mother. I knew my parents had a fine relationship, but I never realized how much my father adored my mother. There was little hint of his admiration and passion in their visible everyday relationship. Only after my mother sank into Alzheimer's did my grief-worn father reveal his immeasurable love. He didn't talk about his feelings: He was, after all, a World War II veteran and a man taught to stoically endure for the sake of his family. But he showed me his devotion every day.

"Isn't she beautiful?" he said to me one day, as we sat with mom in the nursing home's private dining room, sharing a lunch I'd brought: my parents' favorite broccoli soup, half a tuna fish sandwich and a brownie. Mom had a little fleck of mayonnaise-laden tuna on her cheek and a blob of greenish soup on her bib. Her hair was greasy—she'd been resistant to taking a bath. To me, she looked like an old crone from the fairy tales, the kind of dirty, mysterious witch who might whisper a cryptic piece of wisdom that would save your life, but who certainly wouldn't win a beauty contest. I couldn't see what my father saw.

"Your mother looks so pretty in that sweatshirt," my father said a couple of weeks later. We were strolling the corridors of the memory care unit. Mom was shuffling along, holding each of our arms, her head bent. My mother's former wardrobe had gone the way of buttons and zippers and she now wore primarily sweats. I hadn't really noticed her outfit, but I stopped to look. Her pink sweatshirt highlighted the blush of color in her cheeks. When she looked at me and smiled, she might have been wearing a rose chiffon evening gown. Her face glowed. It took my father's observation for me to see my mother in a new light.

"I've discovered a sure-fire way to make your mother smile," my father said, later, when Mom was deep into the advanced stages. We were seated next to Mom's bed, watching her twist her sheet. I scooted forward, eager for my father's insights. My usual ways of making Mom smile were failing me and I felt bereft when she and I were unable to connect.

"Watch this," he said and he leaned forward and gave Mom a series of light kisses on her cheek. She smiled, then she giggled and her beauty shone so strongly that I fully understood what my father had always known: Beauty is there, if you're looking with your heart.

~Deborah Shouse

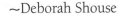

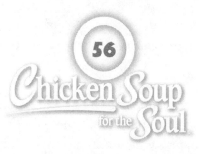

Living in the Moment

Life is a great big canvas, and you should throw all the paint on it you can.
~Danny Kaye

"Well, this doesn't make sense!" For the second month in a row, my husband could not balance our checkbook. Lew had worked in the finance industry for more than fifty years, and numbers were his thing. So for him to have trouble balancing the checkbook was unthinkable. But there it was.

There had been other signs, but how does one know whether they are part of the aging process, or something more serious? Lew was in his early seventies when he started having occasional episodes of transient global amnesia, a temporary loss of memory that passes in a few hours. After the first episode, Lew was tested for a stroke. Included in the tests was an MRI of the brain, and although no stroke was diagnosed, it served as a baseline for later Alzheimer's diagnostic tests.

In retrospect, we realize there were a number of signs related to Alzheimer's. Loss of interest in activities he once enjoyed was one of the more obvious ones. He gradually stopped playing golf with the guys, three times a week slowly dropping to once a week. Participation in an online football pool with good friends and our son had netted Lew some nice winnings, and he liked studying the teams and making his picks. So no one could understand why he decided not to participate anymore and no amount of coaxing by friends and loved ones could change his mind.

After the issue with the checkbook, our family physician referred him to a neurologist, who confirmed the diagnosis of early-stage Alzheimer's disease.

Lew found the diagnosis to be a relief. Now he knew why these odd things had been happening to him. I, on the other hand, went into mourning. I believed his life and ours together was over. I am an organizer and planner by nature. I quickly learned that Alzheimer's disease is not something you can organize or plan. I felt helpless.

The one thing we could do was to learn as much about the disease as possible. During the next six months we spent hours reading everything we could find. We attended workshops offered by the local chapter of the Alzheimer's Association: Help and Hope, The Savvy Caregiver, and The Confident Caregiver Series. Attendance at a local caregiver's support group has been a lifesaver for me. We also participated in a writing workshop so we could tell "Our Love Story."

And we learned to share the diagnosis with family members and friends. The more open we were, the more understanding and support we received. We had been making plans to drop out of our couple's golf traveling group and a number of other social activities. Fortunately, our friends wouldn't hear of it. As they explained, we are all getting older and will have different challenges along the way—and we plan to face them together.

Lew is a pragmatic man with a wonderful sense of humor. He has never denied having the disease and is the first to acknowledge that losing track of strokes on the golf course or not knowing which hole he is playing is because of Alzheimer's.

We have been married for more than forty years and love to travel. When we first received the Alzheimer's diagnosis, we thought our travel days were over and we were fortunate to be able to look back at all the joys experienced in all the countries we had visited and the friends we had made. A couple of months prior to the diagnosis, we took a cruise to Canada and Alaska. Within a short time, Lew didn't remember anything about it. I thought, why spend money on trips he won't remember?

Then we had an "ah-ha" moment. We realized life was not over. That first year following the diagnosis was spent learning, the second we started living our lives again. One day I looked at Lew and realized that it isn't about what he does or doesn't remember—life is really about living in the moment.

During the second year we took some short golf trips, a nineteen-day cruise through the Panama Canal, and two road trips—one to Oregon and another to Sedona, Arizona—all with good friends.

When we were dating we had discovered we both loved to play cribbage, and we like party bridge. Two years post-diagnosis, we still play cribbage every day and bridge often. Lew might not remember the day of the week or the month of the year, but he can still bid and play a great game of cards. And we still play golf, but I have a better chance of beating him now. He prefers playing with me alone or with other couples, instead of with the guys, as that is his comfort level.

Our son recently spent an afternoon videotaping a conversation with his dad about his past, and life in general, as a visual and audio recording for his children. I'm still working on our "Love Story," have finished "Lew's Story," and started "Our Story." We have had such a great life together; we want to share it with our grandsons.

Two years post-diagnosis, Lew's disease has progressed to the point that he can't drive anymore. His response to losing his driver's license was to send out an e-mail to friends and family announcing he is taking applications for chauffeurs. Life is good when you roll with the punches.

One late afternoon we were sitting on the bank of the Rogue River with our friends, watching the fishing and rafting, when Lew turned to me and said, "We are having the best time. I'm sorry I won't be able to remember it." I raised my glass of wine, Lew raised his can of beer, and we toasted to "Living in the Moment."

~Sue Watkins

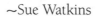

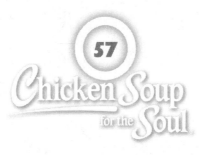

57

The Talk

I have found the paradox that if I love until it hurts, then there is no hurt,
but only more love.
~Mother Teresa

knew something was different about her the moment we first danced at Parents without Partners, a social club for single parents. I felt a disconcerting ridge along her ribcage. I recognized thoracic scoliosis, a curvature of the spine. Fifteen years prior to that eventful evening, I had developed a new type of brace specifically made to treat that condition.

I asked her out for the following Saturday and, just seven days later, I proposed marriage. In a mere six weeks, we were on our honeymoon. By that point, my wife's spinal curvature, to my loving eyes, has so completely disappeared that even now I have to stop and think which side it is on. I loved her just the way she was.

During the past twenty-five years, we've been blessed in so many ways. My wife's three boys, who have matured into wonderful husbands and fathers, are a joy to us both. Their love for their mother and acceptance of me as a stepfather, however strained at first, has given us incredible peace.

We've endured some bumps along the way. An airplane crash, which could have been tragic, left me partially disabled—my arm and hand were paralyzed for half a year. I was broken and depressed until, getting ready for church one Sunday, I was able to move my finger just a quarter of an inch. That day became a turning point in our lives, and with my wife's loving support and my never-give-up attitude, I woke up to the realization that everything was going to be okay.

My last little invention turned into a business that spanned half the globe and allowed a lifestyle that gave us the means to help others in so many ways.

Sometimes, just when you think you've got everything under control, make plans for the future, and are set for new adventure, something intrudes, bringing it all to a screeching halt.

After years of minor memory lapses that gradually became noticeable to family and friends, my wife began having major memory issues. Forgetting how to start a car. Not getting the mail for three days. Asking the same question many times in a row, forgetting appointments and social invitations, paying some bills twice and others not at all, thinking I'd put new tires and wheels on her golf cart... the list goes on.

I needed to communicate my feelings in the kindest, most sensitive manner possible. I started by giving her a beautiful greeting card about love. I'd added words of my own, telling her that, no matter the circumstances, I'd be her man and would love her, care for her, and be by her side forever.

She thanked me through tears, and I led her to the sofa and started The Talk, something I'd been dreading and could no longer put off.

I began by asking her to reminisce about those times I would come into the house, put down a tool I was working with, get a drink and return to the hangar... leaving my tool behind on the counter. We laughed about how I was the absentminded genius, notorious for being scatterbrained. I asked her if I had been a good husband to her for the past twenty-six years and she quipped, "The best one I've had so far." That's my girl.

I held her tightly and, as gently as I could, asked her if she ever had done any research of her own, avoiding saying Alzheimer's. She hadn't and admitted that she was afraid to for fear of what she might learn. Cuddled together, we looked at a few websites, many of which suggested Alzheimer's as the reason for her symptoms. As I scanned the text, hoping she wouldn't notice the "tough parts," she nestled under my arm. That evening, I found her at the computer, pouring over page after page for two hours. I could see stages, no cure, and, of course, the final act. Later that night in bed, I felt her shaking. Reaching to touch her beautiful face, I felt tears.

Turning to me, she posed an even tougher question. "Honey, you're so smart. Will you invent a cure for me?"

"I sure will baby doll, I'll really try," I replied.

Sleepless, the promise I made burning in my brain, I silently made my way down to the workshop. Walking past welders, milling machine, drill press, saws, and testing equipment, I sat at my old workbench, scarred with the tinkerings of past inventions that changed so many lives for the better.

I brushed aside the workings of the "next big thing," and contemplated the pile of cams, gears, springs, and bearings. I picked up one of the gears, examine it for a bit, then spun it on its axle. Like a toy gyroscope, it remained stable for a little while, faltered, then careened off the bench, reminding me of the fragility of her future.

At that moment I realized the awful truth. I'm an inventor, not much more than a glorified mechanic. I can't cure her, I can't help her, and I can't keep my promise.

In the cool dark of the shop, I put my head down, and sobbed myself to sleep.

~Bruce Michael Williams

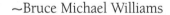

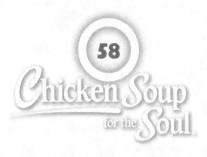

58

Snowflakes and Sunshine

Let us dance in the sun, wearing wild flowers in our hair...
~Susan Polis Shutz

t was a beautiful crisp fall day and I decided my husband Bill and I needed an outing. His Alzheimer's was progressing and some days his world was dark and confusing. Heading out from our home, which is up against the foothills thirty miles west of Denver, we drove along Highway 285 toward the Continental Divide. I had taken on the role of driver without ever really thinking about it. With Bill in the passenger seat and our two Border Collies in the back, we sang to the oldies station as we drove along, enjoying the changing colors of the Aspen trees.

Cresting my favorite pass in Colorado, the valley spread out below us, mountain peaks off in the distance. Bill pointed, and as if seeing it for the first time, tried to tell me how pretty the trees looked. Bill's verbal skills had changed. With friends and family he entered into conversations less frequently and even with me he was having more trouble finding words and putting sentences together.

At Fairplay, we turned north and onto a dirt road to head over Boreas Pass, which would eventually drop us down into Breckenridge. My nephew and his girlfriend were attending college nearby, so our plan was to meet them there for lunch.

As we headed over Boreas Pass, which was lined with Aspens

just dropping their bright yellow leaves, Bill opened his window and stuck his head out to feel the breeze on his face. He suddenly looked over at me and said, "It's snowing."

Sure enough, on this beautiful blue-sky day, it had started to snow. He stuck his head back out the window and opened his mouth to catch the snowflakes. At that moment I knew we had to pull over and enjoy what for Bill was a moment of pure joy. He wasn't thinking about his disease and what it was taking from him, he was living in that moment, capturing snowflakes on his tongue.

I stopped the car and we all got out to stand in the falling snow. It only lasted a few minutes and then the sun shone down once again. I had Bill sit with our dogs, Cody and Raisin, so I could take a picture. It's one I cherish, of a day when the only thing we focused on for one moment was being together with our dogs, in the mountains, in the unexpected snow.

Joining him as time stood still is the most important lesson I learned from our journey with Alzheimer's. Treasure every moment and go wherever that moment takes you with the person you love. There are plenty of dark days, so enjoy the time you are given when those happy moments come along. The sun can definitely shine even while the snow is falling.

~Sara Spaulding

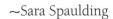

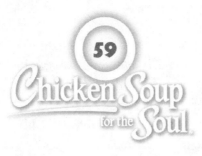

Joy Through Tears

Act as if what you do makes a difference. It does.
~William James

"Hi, my name is Ken. I am living with Alzheimer's disease." This is what my husband says when telling the story of his journey with Alzheimer's. It took more than a year for him to become so forthcoming, but as he immediately adds, "It is such a relief to be able to say that."

For quite some time, I had noticed changes in Ken's personality and behavior, as well as difficulty with problem solving, reasoning, and judgment, particularly involving our finances. One day, Ken announced we had to file for bankruptcy. How was this possible? We went to an attorney, who confirmed Ken's fears. Shortly after, it became apparent that we would have to give up our home. It took the attorney months to unravel our files and financial records.

One day, I saw Ken sitting at the computer, staring at it for what seemed a very long time. He said he couldn't remember how to turn it on. It was then that I realized this wasn't just forgetfulness.

We went to a doctor who specialized in geriatrics. I brought my page-long, typewritten concerns and observations to the appointment. At the bottom of the page I wrote, "Please help us!" The doctor administered tests, and then quietly and calmly stated that my husband had early-stage Alzheimer's disease. An MRI and neuropsychological testing confirmed the diagnosis.

I was relieved, but devastated. Ken was angry and devastated. We had no money, we were going to be homeless, and now we were facing Alzheimer's disease. After speaking with other families living with Alzheimer's, we now know how common financial difficulty, including bankruptcy, can be before a diagnosis.

Within a month we had moved from California to Minnesota to live with our daughter. We stayed with her for six months while we reorganized our lives, but we both continued to be devastated and depressed. Ken was in denial.

A friend called to see how we were doing. I said, "Not well." She suggested I call the Alzheimer's Association on their toll-free 24/7 Helpline (800-272-3900). It provides services to families and professionals, including information, referrals, and care consultation, and it has become what I call my "Lifeline."

When I called the number I was immediately put at ease by a wonderful, warm care consultant, who has continued beside us throughout our journey. Her help, in addition to the support services and educational classes at the Alzheimer's Association, made us realize we had a choice: We could accept what we were facing; or we could remain devastated, fighting the reality of Alzheimer's, which would most assuredly result in more anger, fear, anxiety, and negative energy.

We chose to accept our new now, not to give up, and to have love and compassion for ourselves as well as for others. I started a gratitude journal to celebrate the time Ken and I have together and to recognize his strengths, rather than lament what he is unable to do.

We have learned to live well with Alzheimer's through nutritional eating habits, engaging in social activities, exercising daily and embracing cognitive challenges. We have made music an important part of our lives.

As champions for the fight against Alzheimer's, our lives are purposeful, encouraging, and full of hope. We advocate in our state capital and in Washington, D.C., asking legislators to support research and the Health Outcomes, Planning, and Education (HOPE) for Alzheimer's Act. We speak at Alzheimer's educational events for professionals and families.

Ken is on the Early-Stage Advisory Board for the National Alzheimer's Association and the Minnesota/North Dakota Chapter. He is also a mentor to those who have recently been diagnosed with Alzheimer's through the Peer-to-Peer Outreach Program at our chapter.

Anyone experiencing significant memory problems should see a doctor as soon as possible. Early diagnosis and intervention methods are improving dramatically. Treatment options and sources of support can improve quality of life for the person with the disease, as well as the caregiver and family.

Alzheimer's is not a blessing; but from it many blessings have come to us. I know. I am my love's wife and caregiver. There *is* life after a diagnosis of Alzheimer's. There is joy through tears.

~Mary Margaret Lehmann

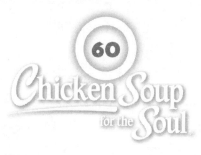

I'll Never Know

As long as I can I will look at this world for both of us.
As long as I can I will laugh with the birds, I will sing with the flowers,
I will pray to the stars, for both of us.
~Sascha, as posted on motivateus.com

had come to visit Ginny. It was our fifty-seventh wedding anniversary.

I could still see that long-ago moment. We stood under the chuppah. I raised my leg and stomped, shattering the glass from which Ginny and I had just sipped the wine of our wedded unity.

But at this moment, she sat stiffly in her lounge chair, at the end of the lineup of skinny old women and frail old men, slouched in their recliners in the community room of the Alzheimer's dementia facility. They looked at the fleeting images and heard the sounds of the soap operas flickering from the new forty-inch flat screen TV.

As I rolled my wheelchair past the residents, my eyes were fixed on Ginny. I stared hard at her face, trying to determine if she, too, remembered that day. Could she still see us standing arm-through-arm before the open arc, the sanctuary of the Torah?

"Hi, Gin, it's me." No response. She stared into space.

"Me, Richie," I said, trying again.

Nothing happened. She didn't move. Her expression didn't change. She showed no awareness of my presence. I said under my breath, "Have you forgotten the sound of my voice?"

Moving my wheelchair closer to her recliner I whispered into her thin white hair, "Your Richie."

I circled from side to side, inching closer, pleading with her to recognize my voice—to know who I was; to be aware of me. But Ginny, her memory of me lost, remained frozen, staring straight ahead.

Finally, I twisted in my chair, bent over, faced her head-on, trying to make eye contact; but it was as if she looked through me. Her eyes were empty, staring at God knows what. Certainly not me, as I shifted to position my eyes right in front of hers.

From within her whitewashed face—a whiteout of expression—her green eyes remained blank. Through the thick lenses of her glasses, her eyes were enlarged, misshapen, like the reflection in a funhouse mirror, distorted and engulfed by large purple, puffy circles.

As I circled around Ginny again, talking softly to her, telling her I love her, reminding her of our house, trying to make her remember walking with our dog, she dropped deeper into the recliner, leaned back against the faded, frayed, and stained maroon upholstery. Her legs popped up onto the equally faded, frayed, and stained footrest. My shoulders sagged in despair. Closing my eyes, I exhaled. And I wondered. How many others had sunk down on this chair and lost themselves in their darkened minds?

Just then, the TV shouted as a caregiver turned up the volume. It was *Guiding Light*. Or *General Hospital*. Or was it *As the World Turns*. What difference did it make? Ivory Soap. Dawn. Spray & Clean. Ring-Around-the-Collar, all flashed by. Whatever!

Nobody watched anyway. They sat like children in kindergarten, waiting for the afternoon movie. Like Ginny, they stared, lost in the meanderings of their minds; or they slept; or they played with their stuffed teddy bears; some caressed cloth babies.

A movie started. "The hills are alive/With the sounds of music." As Julie Andrews sang, heads turned. Chins were raised from chests. People were pulled out of daydreams. But Ginny stared straight and still. Her eyes glazed over as the sounds of music slipped over her expressionless face.

"It's still me—Richie," I softly said, as I lightly touched her shoulder.

Her eyes shifted toward me. Her eyebrows raised. She must have recognized my voice. She moved her lips... I waited. I bent toward her, pulled as if by a magnet, closer, to hear her speak. "What?" I hesitatingly pleaded.

Nothing came out.

No words.

Again I sagged. I was drained.

She furrowed her brow. Frowned. Sucked in her lips. Widened her stare. Grunted. Her face twisted and tightened. She raised her hands and tried to stand. Sitting in my wheelchair, I felt my body trying to rise with her. She wanted to speak, but only emitted sounds from deep in her throat—"Arrgghh! Arrgghh!"

Then it was my turn to stare, to gaze at her twisted face, her widened eyes, her lips pressed hard together—her frustration straining to burst out. My chest pushing out with her.

I said it to myself: What's in your mind? What are you trying to say?

I wanted to hear: I know you! You're my Richie! I love you and have missed you!

Was that it? Was that what she was saying? How could I tell if that's what she was thinking? By her angry face? Her pursed lips? Her guttural noises?

"Tell me," I said, my voice a whisper.

"ARRGGHH!!!"

I'll never know.

~Richard Weinman

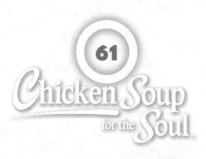

My Mother's Kitchen

When you look at your life, the greatest happinesses are family happinesses.
~Dr. Joyce Brothers

Yesterday when making my weekly bread, I reached for one of my two wooden spoons—the ones I've now used for more than twenty years, and rubbed the smooth wood under my thumb.

I think of my mother's worn wooden spoons and realize I'm recreating her kitchen: the large white mixing bowls, the red wood-handled wire pastry blender. I now have a copy of the silver-topped English jam jar I broke as a child.

I realize my three sisters are doing the same. When we gather in Maine in the summer we head for the collectibles stores and the treasures we find are those we grew up with. One sister collects restaurant ware and casserole dishes from the '50s, another snatches up aged cast iron frying pans, and we all look for the one bowl that will complete our sets of primary-colored Pyrex mixing bowls.

My mother's kitchen is still intact, but now when I visit her in New Hampshire I never know where I'll find these well-loved tools. She has Alzheimer's, and the disease has progressed to the point where putting away the dishes is a frustrating guessing game.

My father has taken over the cooking. We were stunned when we discovered he was watching Emeril. Now he calls to ask me for my johnnycake recipe, and to report on his latest culinary achievement—his quickie pineapple upside-down cake made using the old cast iron pan and (horrors) a cake mix.

This summer he'd call with weekly tallies: quarts of beans frozen, berries picked and turned into jam, reports on the plentiful rhubarb that became sauce, all with a pride we'd never seen before. Previously, all of the work to feed our family of seven was done by my mother.

But it's more than pride I see. It's good caregiving. My mother and father can spend time together in the garden and later in the kitchen because it's familiar to her and safe.

Last summer they were more than regulars at the U-Pick blueberry fields. Their time spent together resulted in blueberry jam. He didn't have to worry about her whereabouts, and conversations over blueberry bushes are always disjointed anyway.

My father has never taken a caregiving class, but he's a remarkable giver of care, and maybe he learned that from my mother. As adults, my sisters and I have always called her for a recipe, for her healthy outrage over our broken hearts, or for her diagnosis of a middle-of-the night malady.

We've lost that now; asking her for the recipe for those brown-sugar pickles we called snakes just causes her frustration. So we don't call her with those questions, and we try to mother each other instead.

My sisters and I continue to recreate my mother's kitchen, surrounding ourselves with the familiar as she becomes a stranger. My kitchen is full. I don't need another cutting board in the shape of a pig. And although the pie-crust-making gene skipped me, not only do I have one red-handled wire pastry blender, I have two.

But now I realize there will never be enough sets of nesting Pyrex mixing bowls in the world to hold our feelings of loss.

~Susan DeWitt Wilder

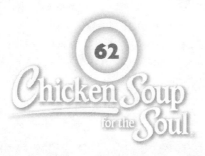

While He Still Remembers

What you need to know about the past is that no matter what has happened,
it has all worked together to bring you to this very moment.

~Author Unknown

My husband and I are alone, for a change, riding home after dropping our kids with their aunt for the night. It's dark and raining, one of those nights when all you can think about is getting home to your warm, cozy house and getting into something comfy.

I have been working on ways to have "quality time" with my husband and this has become more difficult as his Alzheimer's disease progresses. In the dark car, as we drive home, I begin to ask questions about his life in the past. It has occurred to me recently that I know little about that time, as he has always been a person who tends to live "in the now"—not thinking much of the past. But as his life relentlessly slips from his memory, I have been trying to accumulate bits and pieces to share, later, with the family, sure there is so much we don't know.

Tomorrow is Halloween and, thinking this might generate a great story for the grandkids, I ask, "What did you do as a child on Halloween?"

"I don't remember," he replies. "Nothing, I guess," and then slips back into silence.

"Did you ever see a ghost?" I ask.

"No, did you?" he says and quiet sets in again.

"I have!" I shoot into the darkness, and enthusiastically, with great detail, tell him my story. No response.

Finally, he says, "Well, I don't believe in ghosts." It grows quiet again.

Not wanting to give up, I try subject after subject, trying to find something he will bite on; a memory that will spark a good story; a memory he will share. He was always so good at conversation, so interesting, so quick to join in, with enthusiasm, with his opinion on most any subject. But, his answers remain short and hold little to build on, and finally, too disappointed to try anymore, I let the quiet take over.

We ride that way for several miles. Then, out of the darkness he says, "I really like the warm jacket you bought for me today. It's going to be nice and warm this winter." He reaches over and touches my hand. "Thank you," he says softly.

"I'm glad you like it," I reply.

In the now, again, I think, and I wonder how it must be to give so little thought to the past and to live only "in the now." His most consistent question is always to ask, "What day is it today?" As of late, he hardly mentions yesterday. I wonder if he still knows there was a yesterday.

It occurs to me that, as the disease progresses, I will be part of yesterday. I know there will come a time when he will look at me and see a stranger. It's at those times when I wonder: Who will he remember? For now, he still remembers those he sees every day and those he loved most from his past. But the day-to-day stuff barely touches him enough to generate a comment or to commit to memory.

"Thank you for the warm jacket," the touch of his hand in the dark, a connection. This is his world today. I feel an urgent desire to try to prod memories from him before it is too late. I want him to remember childhood laughter and friendships, Christmases past and summers gone by. I want him to remember the melodies of the gospel songs he once sang and loved and I want to hear him sing them again.

I want him to remember the night we first kissed under the stars. But, he doesn't. He smiles when I tell him about that night. But, it's like a nice story he once heard and he's happy I remember. I was hoping for more. I need so much more.

We pull into the driveway and turn off the car. We sit in the darkness for a moment. "It's nice to be home," he says, quietly. I get out of the car and the motion light goes on. He gets out and, without another word, shuffles into the house. I follow slowly, smiling to see he has worn his new jacket.

He is happy. He is happy right now at this moment. I guess that is what matters. And that, for right now, he still remembers.

~Susan Hanna Frook

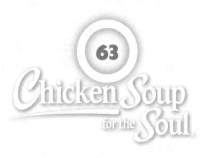

The Power of What Is

The larger the island of knowledge, the longer the shoreline of wonder.
~Ralph W. Sockman

I pressed the phone against my ear, not wanting to miss a word the doctor said. "The PET scan was affirmative for Alzheimer's," his voice matter-of-fact.

The doctor explained how both hemispheres of the brain have five lobes, and while my husband Ray had plaque in four of them, there was none found in the frontal lobes. This meant he would still have the skills related to attention, planning, and motivation.

Odd as it might sound, this information thrilled me. I knew from his primary care physician's diagnosis, and Ray's increasing confusion in many areas of his life, that he had Alzheimer's. These new facts would help me be a better caregiver.

I approached caregiving in much the same way I had approached parenting my young children. When I ran into problems while rearing them, I pulled out my books on child development and looked up the characteristics of a child at a given age. I could then adjust my expectations and requirements, and make both of us feel better. I called it the power of "What Is."

Based on what the doctor told me, for now Ray still the skills necessary to pack his backpack with what he needed for his weekly art class at the Alzheimer's Association; or make a short grocery list, walk to the store, and buy what he wanted.

"Can he really pack his own backpack?" other caregivers asked. "Aren't you worried he'll get lost when he walks to the store?"

"He can still organize his things. And he wears a MedicAlert + Alzheimer's Association Safe Return bracelet," I told them. "He walks all over our neighborhood and never gets lost."

But he couldn't do other things our friends with Alzheimer's could do. I was deep in thought about my conversation with the doctor when Ray walked in wearing old, baggy sweat pants; a crisp, new short-sleeved dress shirt; and the brown felt hat he'd taken to putting on in any kind of weather.

I looked at my husband. Comfort was now one of his greatest concerns, and my concerns had grown much more serious than clothing. Making sure he wasn't going to be too warm or too cold was what mattered.

"Let's get going. I'm hungry," Ray urged. Recently I'd noticed him having more trouble coping as evening approached. I'd heard how many people with Alzheimer's had increased difficulties in the evening. There was even a name for it: sundowning. Ray's anxiety could swell into a tidal wave washing over our house if I pushed him when he was tired and his confusion greater. I grabbed the car keys and we headed out for dinner.

When we got to the restaurant Ray pulled out his reading glasses, but didn't look at the menu. "What are you having?" he asked.

Before Alzheimer's took over our lives I hadn't realized how much memory is involved in selecting a meal. I look at an item on the menu, picture the food in my head, and remember whether I like it or not. I had just opened the menu when Ray stood up and headed for a neighboring table.

"Whatever those people next to us are having looks good. I want to ask them what it is," he explained when I took his arm and settled him back in his chair.

A few days earlier we'd had lunch with another couple from our Alzheimer's support group and I'd run into the same embarrassing situation while her husband sat quietly in his chair. The wife had said mildly, "I just order for both of us."

Ray's restaurant behavior was quite new and I searched for the requisite skill to handle it. "You like Pad Thai. I can order that for you," I offered.

Ray nodded, looking relieved. I made a mental note to follow this method from now on. If I eliminated the confusion for him by responding to appropriate expectations, we could enjoy these moments of companionship.

As soon as we got home we started our evening ritual. We put our large calendar out on the kitchen table, like the one I had used for lesson planning when I taught high school. Ray drew an X through the day drawing to a close.

"I have my Kaiser class tomorrow," he said. I wrote "Kaiser class" on a yellow pad labeled "Ray's day."

"I can print off directions for the bus from here to Kaiser," I offered.

"I remember how to get there," he said. "And I have directions from before."

"Let's get them out."

Ray had been attending a weekly class on managing anxiety for several years, but could no longer drive and was becoming surprisingly adept at using the bus system—as long as there was only one transfer and I provided him with written directions. He enjoyed the people he met along the way, and didn't mind if he headed in the wrong direction occasionally. He would ask questions of the driver or passengers until he somehow righted himself. Plus he had his Safe Return bracelet.

"There's an 8:10 bus," he said, looking at the directions. "I'd better get up at 5:00."

"You don't need that much time," I said gently. "That's three hours." Numbers could do tricky things in his head.

"6:00, then."

"Or 6:30," I suggested. I knew when his alarm went off he would probably get right up and head for the shower. But sometimes he turned the alarm off and went back to sleep, having no memory of it going off when I woke him. So right now I was his backup alarm.

Setting expectations for Ray isn't easy. Once I understood what to expect and how to respond, we would have a fairly smooth time for a while, and then what he was able to do would change.

But we are managing, and sometimes even thriving, day by day, as I pay close attention to, and plan around, "What Is."

~Samantha Ducloux Waltz

When you talk with other
caregivers, share your emotions.
Cry and laugh together.
Don't limit conversations to
caregiving tips.

"Ways to cope with grief and loss"

alz.org/care

Chapter 8

Living with Alzheimer's & Other Dementias

The Lighter Side

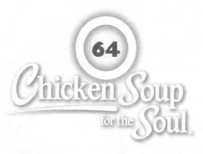

Talking Potato

Common sense and a sense of humor are the same thing,
moving at different speeds. A sense of humor is just common sense, dancing.
~William James

Being creative while taking care of my mom during her last year was not only helpful, but an absolute necessity. As the dementia progressed, she didn't say much and mostly stayed on the couch watching TV.

Eventually, getting her to eat became a challenge. Usually the only thing she wanted was a baked potato with butter and cheese.

One day, after fixing her potato, I headed into the living room, only to hear, "I don't want it."

"I have your potato fixed with butter and cheese. It looks delicious, Mom."

"I don't want it!"

"You are going to love it. It will taste good."

"I don't want it! I don't want anything!"

Mom weighed less than 100 pounds and needed to eat.

"Mr. Potato," I said, "Mom says she doesn't want you."

In another voice I replied, "Tell her I taste good and I want her to eat me."

Mom again, "I don't want him."

"But I'm all covered with butter and cheese and just the right temperature."

Mom's head came up a little, but she kept her eyes closed.

"Tell Betty I will cry if she doesn't eat me!"

Mom's body started jiggling with laughter. She cracked a smile and opened her eyes, looked at me, and said, "Tell him I'll eat him!"

And she did!

As I approached the kitchen to fetch my talking potato, I was thrilled she was going to eat and that I had made her laugh, amazed at what I heard come out of my mouth, and so sad about my mom and her condition—all at the same time.

Later that night my thoughts returned to years earlier when I went to the hospital to visit Mom. As I walked through the door of her room, she said, "I prayed all day that you'd come and see me because I knew if you did, you would make me laugh."

Those words changed my life. I knew I was supposed to use my quick wit and sense of humor to help others and I became a Christian humor writer. Now all these years later I was using humor to help my elderly mother.

Even with dementia she knew there was something funny about a talking potato.

~Linda Rose Etter

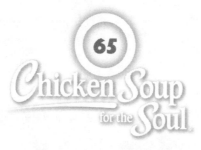

The Soft Side of Alzheimer's

Humor is just another defense against the universe.
~Mel Brooks

have been blessed by having had a wonderfully loving and generous mother-in-law, Fran. Fran has always loved people, cooking and partying, but has always disliked cats.

One day, when we had taken Fran back to her mobile home, she opened the door and a small cat darted from under the front steps and ran inside. Fran began chasing and screaming at the cat, frightening the poor thing half to death! I was finally able to convince Fran to shut herself into the bedroom at the other end of the home while I coaxed the cat out of hiding and got it outside.

Several years later, after Fran had been diagnosed with Alzheimer's disease, I had a shock when I brought Fran to visit a friend of mine one afternoon. I knew my friend had a cat, but the cat generally hid when company came over, so I didn't worry too much about it. While we were sitting in the living room, the cat, a large Maine coon, came out of the bedroom and walked directly over to Fran, rubbing itself against Fran's legs.

I held my breath, waiting for her to scream. Instead, Fran bent over, patted the cat and said, "What a nice dog." That day,

Alzheimer's was Fran's friend, saving her from what might have been a very unpleasant visit.

~Tamera Leland

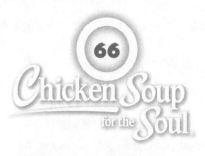

The Bird

*Good manners are just a way of showing other people that
we have respect for them.*
~Bill Kelly

irst there was a knock on my bedroom door. Then my
mother's voice called out: "Jean, there's a bird in my
bathroom." Before my husband, Doyle, or I had time to
respond, Mom appeared like an apparition at the foot of
our bed. "Come quickly," she said. "You've got to get it out."

Doyle pretended to be asleep. I peered over the top of the covers
that were pulled to my chin. In the semi-darkness I could see my
eighty-four-year-old mother's eyes ablaze with conviction. Her short
white hair stood on end, spiking off at irregular angles. She wore a
light summer nightgown, inside out, backward and slightly askew. I
wanted to cry.

Mom lived with us because she had early-stage Alzheimer's
disease. We had grown accustomed to her quirks: the searing hot
Florida days when she applied layer upon layer of clothing to her frail
body, the storing of canned goods and buttered garlic bread under
her pillow, the repetitive questions. But a hallucination caught me
by surprise. That was enough to send me under the pillow, at once
trembling in fear and denial.

"Mom," I said, "birds can't get in the house." This was an eighty-
eight-degree September day. We never opened the windows. Our air
conditioning hummed twenty-four hours a day.

"Je-e-an." Her hands went to her hips; her chest rose and expanded.

I cleared my throat, hoping that would clear my head. "He won't hurt anything," I said. "We'll get him out in the morning."

"Je-e-an." She was accustomed to being in charge, like the fourth grade teacher she had been for thirty years.

Arguing seemed pointless. A bird was in her bathroom—a windowless, second-floor room with a skylight that did not open, a room entered only through her bedroom—and she wanted that bird out *now*. Her face wore a look that, even with her teeth out, said she was not leaving my room until I followed her out.

I slid out of bed and down the worn oak floors in the hallway, into her darkened bedroom. "There's no bird here," I said.

"In the bathroom." She pointed to the door. "Go look."

I stepped into the bathroom. My eyes struggled to adjust to the bright lights that only illuminated the dreadful floral wallpaper I had regretted choosing the moment the paste dried.

No bird. I checked the shower, behind the toilet, under the sink. "Maybe you had a dream, Mom."

"I know what I saw." She pointed to the skylight. "Right there. A bird was flapping around, trying to get out."

"Well, I guess he made it." I clapped. "Good for him. Can we go to bed now?"

Mom hung her head and wrung her hands. "I know you think I'm crazy," she said. The smartest woman I'd ever known looked bewildered and close to tears.

Guilt over being too flippant weighed on my conscience and pulled my shoulders into a slump. I turned my weary self back into her bedroom and looked up to the heavens for guidance.

From the top of the armoire across her room, a huge black bird looked back. "Whoa!" I screamed.

To my stunned eyes, the bird appeared the size of a giant condor. I threw my arms around Mom, although she showed no sign of needing my protection. She drew in a breath that raised her shoulders all the way to her ears, then sighed relief, like a witch whose burning had been called off when her visions proved to be true.

The grackle, in reality about a foot high, took wing. Black, iridescent plumage glistened in the low light as the bird zigged, then zagged over our heads. Panic glued my feet to the floor, my hands to my mother.

The sounds and smells of fear must have jolted our cat, Ray, from his nap on the first-floor sofa. Little padded feet pounded up the wooden steps, then galloped full speed down the hall and into Mom's room.

Swoop! The bird found the door. Screech! Ray ground to a stop, jumped in the air and reversed course. The bird, the cat, and the panicked daughter flew, raced and bumbled our way out of the room, along the hall and down the stairs. At the bottom, I turned to see Mom gliding behind, head held high.

The terrified bird careened around the kitchen, seeking an escape. I sped to open the back door where I stood like a flight attendant, pointing to the exit, wishing I could whistle to get the bird's attention, failing to see the imminent danger posed by Ray. After all, cats can't fly, I reasoned, as Ray jumped onto the kitchen counter and soared into space. Snap! He caught the bird in his jaws mid-air. Plop! Ray landed. The bird hung in limp clumps of black out of either side of his mouth. Out the door they went.

Doyle arrived in the kitchen. "What is going on?"

"You'll think I'm crazy," I said. Mom and I laughed.

"What's so funny?"

"A bird was in the house," I said.

Doyle rubbed his chin and regarded me with suspicion.

And for one enlightening moment, I imagined how desperate I would feel if my husband didn't believe me, if he second-guessed everything I said or did.

When my children and friends called in the morning, I spun elaborate versions of Mom's triumph. She pressed against me, soaking in every word as I told of her patient effort to make me see. Mom knew she was losing control over her life, giving up her freedom and her home, but she seemed to find comfort in believing that we still listened to her and trusted her judgment.

Rather than a harbinger of death, our black-plumed visitor served to remind me that my primary mission in caring for Mom was not to prevent her dying, but to preserve the dignity of her life.

~Jean Salisbury Campbell

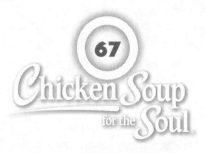

67

Laughter Through the Tears

Every survival kit should include a sense of humor.
~Author Unknown

As a group facilitator for caregivers of people living with Alzheimer's disease, we struggled through some very intense moments at our weekly meetings together. As each person related her personal story, the atmosphere of sadness was palpable. The saving grace for our group were those moments of humor that cut through the shared sorrow.

This afternoon, group had been especially painful. One woman grieved over the seeming injustice of life. Her husband had been a brilliant physicist and now he didn't know how to get dressed. Another member was sick with worry when her mom somehow wandered away from home and was lost for hours. Frankly, it was an emotionally exhausting session.

The last to share her story was "Evelyn," whose husband was stricken with the disease fairly early in life. She began sort of hesitantly, looking as though maybe her experience was not appropriate to share. "My problem, I guess, is unusual," she said, nervously. "This is about our sexual relations. Is it okay to talk about it?"

I assured her that what is said here, stays here. Then I added, "As long as the issue is related to your husband's struggle with Alzheimer's disease and you are comfortable with it, go ahead."

"Well my husband has always had a strong sex drive. He had it when he was healthy and he has it now." She paused. "The problem is that now his short-term memory is gone." One of the group interrupted Evelyn. "So how does his loss of memory affect him? Like he has forgotten how to have sex?"

"Good grief, no," exclaimed Evelyn. "The problem is that we will have sex in the morning and by lunchtime he forgets that we had sex. He will approach me longingly and say 'Honey, c'mon, we haven't had sex for days.' He is insatiable."

For what seemed like an eternity, there was silence. I was trying to think of something appropriate to say, but for the life of me, I couldn't.

Evelyn blushed. "I shouldn't have brought it up," she said.

Then from the other side of the room, I heard a suppressed laugh. Evelyn at first looked askance at the offender. Then someone else tittered. Evelyn herself started to laugh.

Before you knew it, our professional group had lost all restraint, breaking into unrestrained laughter. I tried to regain control. "Oh, Evelyn I'm sorry, that must be…"

"Wonderful?" interrupted one woman. Another piped up with, "I wish my George had that problem." Other semi-ribald remarks followed, with Evelyn, by this time, bent over with laughter.

I don't remember if we ever solved Evelyn's problem that day, but I do know that the cloud of depression that had hung over us was gone. Despite our pain, we found we could laugh at ourselves. The laughter had broken through our despair, as we passed around the box of Kleenex to dry our tears of laughter.

~Hank Mattimore

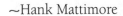

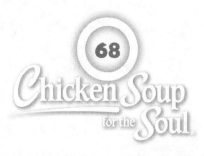

68

French Toast

Mirth is God's medicine. Everybody ought to bathe in it.
~Henry Ward Beecher

ospital stays are never easy, but they are even more difficult for someone with Alzheimer's. My dad spent two weeks in the hospital recuperating from surgery. Attempts at physical rehab were not going well because he was unable to understand instructions, let alone follow them. The nurses had to guess at his pain management, because he was not reliably able to communicate how he was feeling. He remained bed-ridden, sleeping most of the time. His appetite was poor, despite my mom's best attempts at coaxing him to eat.

One morning, a surly worker from the hospital kitchen shuffled into my dad's room. He clearly was not happy about his job, his life, or both.

"Scrambled eggs and bacon, oatmeal with fruit, or French toast." The hospital staffer sighed and waited to check the box by the meal option Dad selected. Dad remained mute and Mom thought she was going to have to make a selection for him.

Suddenly Dad perked up. He had an important question.

"Does the French toast speak French?"

The hospital worker broke into a wide grin that seemed to brighten the whole room. He shot my mom a mischievous look.

"It sure does."

So Dad ordered the French toast, while my mom laughed with the hospital employee, who was no longer surly.

One of the last lucid things my dad told me before he sank deep into the grips of Alzheimer's was that you need to keep your sense of humor.

He was so right.

~Joy Johnston

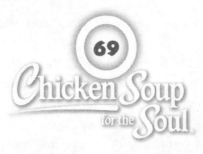

Comic Relief

Humor is merely tragedy standing on its head with its pants torn.
~Irvin S. Cobb

After two years of caregiving for my mom, I learned to be with her in the present—or past. Asking her what she had for lunch did not work. She couldn't remember. Complimenting her on the craft items she had made earlier in the week did not work either. She thought someone else had made them.

I also learned not to fight a losing battle. There is no point disagreeing with someone who is passionate about something. It's better to enter their world and solve the problem for them… in their reality, not in yours.

And finally, it's important to let yourself laugh. There were plenty of laughs along the way in the assisted living complex where Mom lived during those two years. I felt a twinge of guilt laughing at the behaviors and remarks of the residents, but as friends would often remind me, "You either laugh or you cry."

One of the aides once asked Carrie, a ninety-eight-year-old resident, if she was ready to go into the dining room for dinner, and she replied, "Oh no, I can't do that. My mother is coming by this afternoon."

Elsie, a resident with Alzheimer's who frequently sat in the lobby, reached up to me one day from her wheelchair and whispered, "Did you get an invitation to the party?"

I hesitated, not knowing how to respond, then answered, "No, did you?"

She slumped in her chair and said, "No."

I leaned in and whispered, "I'll find out who *is* invited and let you know. How would that be?" Her eyes lit up and she gave me a high five. Felt like high school all over again.

My mom cracked me up every now and then, too. When I told her my best friend from high school was coming to town for our fiftieth high school reunion, she leaned in and grinned. "Does Shirley know you're old?"

One day during craft hour, I sat with Mom helping her color a page with clowns on it. A dozen or so of us were sitting around a large table with bowls of Magic Markers on it. The ladies were laughing and teasing while coloring, freely using the markers before tossing them back into the bowls. Except for Roxie.

The activities director leaned over Roxie's shoulder and asked, "Why aren't you coloring, Roxie?" Roxie turned to the director and said, flat out, "I can't use these markers. They're for left-handed people!" I had to stifle myself on that one.

Ginny caught my arm one day as I entered the facility demanding to know if I had stolen her clothes. When I told her no, she screamed, "Liar!"

I told her maybe I could help her find them. Together we walked hand-in-hand to her room and opened the closet door. It was full. "There, Ginny," I said, "Your clothes are back where they belong. Isn't that great?" She reached over and gave me a bear hug.

I was proud that I was learning to enter the world of these individuals instead of looking at things from my vantage point. I had to accept the fact that my mom, because of her short-term memory loss, had become someone else. And, because of that, I, too, had to become someone else.

Then there was Margie, who rushed into the office one day wringing her hands, on the verge of tears, begging, "I need help; I've lost January." I had overheard the remark sitting in the lobby, and wondered how the director would handle that one. The executive director got up from her chair, came rushing around her desk and grabbed Margie, saying, "Let's go to your room." A few minutes later she returned with the story. Margie had turned over the page in her calendar that read December and there was no January page. Margie was promised a new calendar. Problem solved with finesse.

Most of those dear souls have passed away, including my mom. Others were sent to nursing homes; a few to other facilities. But all left an impression on those of us who were left behind.

~Rosemary Barkes

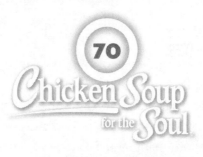

Armchair Shopper

A bargain is something you can't use at a price you can't resist.
~Franklin P. Jones

I n the beginning, we didn't realize what was happening. We weren't sure if Grandma Doris was just forgetful, or if it was deeper than that. She'd forget to eat lunch or she'd eat it twice. She'd forget to check her mail for a week or two at a time. She'd forget that she had already fed her dog, Feisty, and feed him again (several times a day).

But the last straw was when she put a cake in the oven, engaged the safety latch and then forgot how to open it. That cake baked until it turned black and smoked filled her apartment and the fire department was called. My parents decided she should move in with them.

Dad took Grandma Doris's driver's license away, so she had to depend on us to get around. Oh boy, did she love to shop! She could peruse every aisle of every store for hours. She would inevitably come home with something that she just couldn't live without.

Whenever I made a trip to my dad's, I always asked Grandma if she wanted a ride to go shopping, which she usually did. Over time, as her Alzheimer's progressed, her excitement for shopping lessened. Sad, I thought. She must be losing her spunk. Over dinner one weekend, I told my parents I was concerned that Grandma no longer seemed to want to go shopping. It seemed like she wasn't herself anymore. To the contrary, they explained. Grandma was doing great. In fact, she was shopping more than ever.

Grandma, they told me, had discovered the home shopping channel. Everything she could ever want, she could find in the comfort of her own room, while lounging on her navy blue tweed recliner. I sat with her one day and observed her as she watched the shopping channel. She was captivated by the hosts. She held onto every word they said about colors, materials, sizes, shapes, quality, customer reviews, and testimonials. Sure enough, if she liked an item, she'd pick up the phone and order it right then and there. She had no idea what she needed it for, or what she'd do with it, but that didn't matter. She never put her credit card away—she just kept it out, next to the phone, just in case.

The next time I came to visit, my parents gave me an update and told me all was well. She was still watching the shopping channel but was ordering items less frequently. It seemed harmless, so they didn't stop her, especially because it made her happy and gave her a sense of freedom.

The next morning, the deliveryman came to the door with a rather large box. My parents joked with the man, (who they knew rather well by now) and wondered what Grandma had ordered that was so large and heavy. He said there were six more just like this box in the truck. He loaded the rest of them on his handcart and wheeled them up to the door. We thanked him and away he went.

Dad called up to Grandma and told her that her latest shipment was here. My dad opened one as we all stood around with great anticipation. Grandma had no memory of what she had ordered. Packing tape, Styrofoam and a few plastic bags later, Dad pulled a word processor out of the box. It was one of those original word processors from the 1980s—half computer, half typewriter—the latest technology at the time. And there were six more just like it.

Not only did Grandma not know what to do with a word processor, with her arthritic hands, she couldn't type if she wanted to. The four of us stood in the entryway with seven heavy boxes stacked up around us. All we could do was laugh.

After a gentle discussion with Grandma, who still had no recollection of ordering those seven word processors, Dad decided she could no longer have unlimited unsupervised access to her credit card. She could watch the shopping channel, but she would need to ask Dad before she ordered anything.

The shopping channel took all seven word processors back without any problem. The usual deliveryman came to pick them up, and after that, they didn't see as much of him, because Grandma's shopping sprees were curtailed.

Grandma is gone now. The end of her life was hard and sad. But my parents and I try to focus on the funny things. It makes it a little less painful. And to this day, we still chuckle when we think of the word processors.

~Crescent LoMonaco

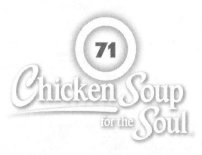

The Bear

The most wasted of all days is that in which we have not laughed.
~Nicolas Chamfort

"Come home *right now*. There's a *bear* in the back yard!"

That's how it all began for us — a sunny day in June that changed everything. The phone in Dad's office rang and it was Mom, matter-of-factly stating there was a bear in our yard. Odd, because in the nearly forty years we had lived in that house, we had never, ever, seen a bear in the yard. We had never even seen a bear in our state!

Dad initially tried to explain to Mom that she didn't have anything to worry about because it couldn't possibly be a bear. She was adamant, however, so he relented and drove home from the office to see what the heck was going on.

When Dad arrived in our driveway, he encountered a massive brown *cow* — standing in our back yard. And my petite, beautiful, seemingly healthy mom, defiantly standing at the back door, hands on her hips, saying, "I *told you* there was a *bear* in the back yard!"

Apparently a cow had escaped from the farm down the road and found her way to our back yard. To this day, I still don't know why Mom saw a bear instead of a cow. But I'm a lot more educated in the symptoms of Alzheimer's now than I was in 2009, so I know that to her, it was a bear. In the years that have passed since then, she never backed down from her conviction. For some reason, she always remembered the bear.

That day was the beginning of a three-year journey into Alzheimer's that tested our perfect little family unit—Mom, Dad and me (a slightly spoiled only child)—in ways we couldn't have imagined. We managed our way through a lot of memories lost. We learned to unplug the oven and hide the car keys. We learned to look in the freezer when the TV remote went missing. We learned to navigate a plethora of drugs and buy sippy cups. We learned that chocolate pudding makes you feel better because, well, it just does. We learned to slow down, sit still, and enjoy one another's company while we still had time. And we laughed. We found great comfort in the fact we could still laugh together no matter what.

Mom passed in 2012. And when people ask me about my family's journey with Alzheimer's, I think it shocks them when I laugh out loud and smile. Not the reaction they expect, I think. Probably not the reaction they get when they ask others that question about this terrible disease.

Then I share the bear story. And they laugh with me. Because Mom forgot where the forks were in the kitchen, she forgot how to put her clothes on, she forgot her sisters, but she never forgot that bear. And any time I asked her about it, right up until the end, she would always tell me the whole story—over and over again—and we would laugh. Out loud. And the only thing that mattered at that point was that it was a memory. And there weren't many of those left—so we cherished it.

~Lisa R. Richardson

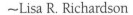

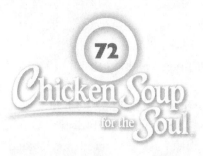

A Mother's Help

God could not be everywhere, so he created mothers.
~Jewish Proverb

My dad continued living in his home of forty years after we moved Mom to a secured dementia assisted living center. One Saturday, I decided to take my mom with me on the seventy-five-mile trip to check on my dad and their house. At this stage, Mom enjoyed riding and being outside. Plus, I knew how much the visit would mean to my dad.

We had a great day together: We enjoyed a meal at the kitchen table, got all the bills paid and mailed, laundry done and put away, the house was fresh and clean, and we made plenty of meals for Dad to enjoy throughout the week.

It was time for Mom and me to head back. Leaving Dad like this was always difficult for me. I knew he wanted us to stay longer, or even to have Mom return home permanently. We both knew that wasn't possible. I always fought back tears as I said goodbye.

We got Mom in the car and safely buckled in. Dad thanked me over and over again for the help. I knew he was grateful for the visit, and I promised him that we would come back again soon. Then we drove off.

Mom entertained me with stories and anything that she could see from her window. I listened quietly as I was pretty exhausted. Then, less than half a mile from Mom's facility, I drove through a green light at the intersection—or at least that would be my story when the red and blue lights flashed behind me.

I pulled over and explained to Mom that this would only take a second. By now, she was seeing a marvelous light show reflecting off the front windshield. Red. Blue. Red. Blue. Totally fascinated, she never noticed the officer approaching my car or the conversation between us. The officer asked where I was headed and I told him my mother lived at the facility nearby and I was taking her back there.

Fortunately, he was all too familiar with the facility because the police station was just two driveways east. Occasionally, some of the residents would get access to a phone and place emergency calls. These calls would soon to be followed by a visit from an officer responding to a call from someone claiming to be "kidnapped."

When he asked for my driver's license and registration I explained that my billfold was in the trunk because Mom had a tendency to take things out of it and hide them, but if he didn't mind I would get it for him. He agreed. I jumped out of my seat and headed to the rear of the car. But when I got there and tried to raise the hatch, the door was locked. I returned to the driver's door, where luckily I had left the window open, to unlock it. Again, I got to the hatch door and again it was locked. Starting to panic, I said to the officer, "Let me try again. I know I unlocked it."

After the third try, the officer suggested that maybe Mom was locking the door as I walked to the hatch. I couldn't hear it because our cars were still running. He said he would hit the unlock button once I got to the back of the car. He was right. As soon as she heard the unlocking sound, my mom would hit the button on the driver's side door, which locked all doors.

Both the officer and I could not contain ourselves. We laughed so hard and shook our heads. What else could we do? He saw the embarrassment and stress on my face. He was so patient and understanding. He simply asked me to be careful because drivers often have bad accidents at that intersection. He told me to take care and offered a blessing for the huge responsibility I had. I expressed my heartfelt appreciation for his understanding and promised to heed his advice.

Within the next sixty seconds, I had Mom back at her place, safe and sound. I headed home to enjoy the alcoholic beverage of my choice and to reflect on yet another moment that would make me laugh and smile for many days to come.

~Cheryl Edwards-Cannon

Music and art can enrich the lives of people with Alzheimer's disease. Both allow for self-expression and engagement, even after dementia has progressed.

"Music, Art and Alzheimer's"

alz.org/care

Chapter
9

Living
with Alzheimer's
& Other Dementias

New Ways to
Make Connections

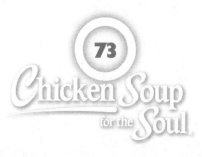

Dancing Words

I see dance being used as communication between body and soul,
to express what is too deep to find for words.
~Ruth St. Denis

As a newly transplanted nursing home administrator in the spring of 1980, I was excited to meet the residents at Phoenix Mountain Nursing Center, a skilled nursing home that had just opened a year earlier. Going from room to room introducing myself and trying to remember each resident's name, I instantly recognized the gentleman I had just met—Mr. Russell Lyon, Sr. I had noticed the large billboards advertising the Russ Lyon Realty Company when house hunting.

I asked if he was a relative, but received a blank stare in return. His nurse confirmed that the well-dressed gentleman I just met was, indeed, the same Mr. Lyon that owned the Russ Lyon Realty Company.

Over the next several months I saw Mr. Lyon daily, usually at lunch or dinner in the dining room. Always impeccably dressed, he never responded to the usual pleasantries of the staff or other residents. The blank stare was always present. Physically, he could walk without assistance and was always compliant with the directions and care provided by the nursing staff.

As Christmas approached, groups came by to sing carols, but the highlight of the holiday season was the evening orchestra presentation a week before Christmas Day. Scheduled almost a year in advance, a well-known orchestra was set to perform in front of a dining room filled to capacity. A thirty-by-thirty-foot dance floor was assembled, wassail and dessert were ready, and families were arriving to take Christmas photos with their loved ones before the show.

The show began with traditional carols, and then the orchestra started playing big band tunes. Mr. Lyon immediately stood, turned to his caregiver, and said, "Would you care to dance?"

The caregiver was astonished but said, "I'd love to." Hand-in-hand they walked to the dance floor and Mr. Lyon began dancing as if he had been practicing just for this event. As he danced he chatted with the staff, said hello, told them that he appreciated the little things that they did for him daily, and that he was frustrated with his inability to communicate with them.

I talked with him during a dance and he told me "I'm still here." While the music played, he danced with all of the nurses and was animated in his discussions—and when the music stopped, the blank stare returned as if a switch had been thrown.

This turn of events was shared with his physician and his family, and we speculated how we could continue to open this channel of communication with Mr. Lyon on a routine basis. A portable cassette player with musical recordings from the 1940s provided the key. Using this method, we were able to continue communicating with Mr. Lyon for another eight months, until the brain cells that controlled that channel of communication for Mr. Lyon quit functioning, too. He died a month later.

Our discovery with Mr. Lyon gave us all a renewed sense of optimism when providing care to others with similar diagnoses because, in our minds, they "were still there," even though normal communication routes were not functioning. Since that time, I have seen similar instances of individuals with Alzheimer's who can communicate through music, art, and, I'm convinced, divine intervention—and I continue to remember what Mr. Lyon said: "I'm still here."

~John White

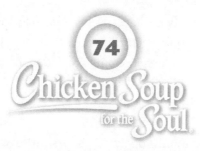

A Bright Spot in Darkness

Animals are such agreeable friends—they ask no questions,
they pass no criticisms.
~George Eliot

It was a Walmart shopping trip I won't forget, because the list was items for my father, who had just been admitted to the long-term care center in our small southern Illinois town. A year earlier, Mom and I had been told that Daddy was in the middle stage of Alzheimer's disease. Two months later, he started to rapidly deteriorate, not just mentally, but also in his mobility. We could see he wanted to stand and walk but his brain couldn't transmit the message to his legs.

My mother, who was ill through much of their marriage, struggled to care for Daddy in their home. Caregivers helped for part of each day, and neighbors checked on my parents as needed. But it became increasingly clear that Daddy was reaching the point where he needed 24/7 professional care. So that day we helped Daddy into the car for his trip to the care center and now I was tearing up as I looked for things to make him comfortable.

Suddenly an idea popped into my head, sending me scurrying to the toy aisle. And there it was. The perfect gift for Daddy. The cutest, softest, cuddliest, stuffed black-and-white dog. What a perfect companion for Daddy to have by his side. He loved his dogs and would miss them. So I hoped this stuffed one would help.

Talk about an understatement! My dad's face lit up when I gave him his new companion and he promptly named him Artie after a good friend. It didn't take long before Artie was the talk of the care center.

Resting comfortably on Daddy's lap, Artie went almost everywhere with Daddy in his wheelchair. They attended church services and other activities. Artie would keep watch at Daddy's bedside when he slept, sometimes sitting by him and other times snuggled under the covers in Daddy's arms.

Because Daddy always wore his Coast Guard cap, my friend Sheryl surprised him on his birthday with a matching cap for Artie. He wore it all the time.

Of course, the dapper pooch also got in trouble. One day, I was in the elevator with Daddy, Artie, and one of the nurse's aides, Lisa. The first thing Lisa said was, "Artie bit me today." I looked at Daddy and asked him if that were true. He smiled as he helped Artie "attack" Lisa's arm again.

Another time I ran into the same trio and Lisa told me, "Artie wet the bed this morning." Daddy grinned and whispered to Artie that it was okay.

Daddy still loved to eat, especially snacks, which he would always share with Artie. One could see by all the cookie crumb stains on Artie's mouth.

During a celebration of "Senior Citizen Month" the care center hired a professional photographer to shoot portraits of residents and families. Daddy, Mom, and I lined up, and on Daddy's lap sat "super model" Artie. That simple stuffed pooch brought so many smiles to our faces as we watched Daddy diminish, disappearing deeper into the disease. What could have been sad, painful visits were brightened by Daddy's smile at Artie's antics.

Nine months after Daddy entered the care center, he passed away. Artie was in bed with him. And he was still sitting guard when

I walked into the room to tell Daddy goodbye before the hearse took him away. I left the care center that day with Artie in my arms.

And there he was at the funeral, a dapper little dog wearing a Coast Guard cap, sitting on a white stool, guarding Daddy's casket.

Artie now sits on a shelf in my home next to many of Daddy's WWII things, under a painting of his farm. I remember all the joy Artie brought Daddy, Mom, and me in the midst of Daddy's battle with Alzheimer's. And I thank God for nudging me that day in the store to buy a stuffed dog, for there is no question about it — Artie was a bright light for us and for my father during the darkness of Alzheimer's.

~Linda Veath Cox

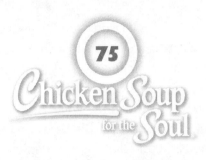

75

My Ticket to Happiness

All great artists draw from the same resource: the human heart,
which tells us that we are all more alike than we are unalike.
~Maya Angelou

When I was a young girl my dad called me "Ticket." I don't know how old I was when I asked him why he called me that, but I remember the answer. He told me that I was his "Ticket to Happiness." That name made me feel special and wanted. It made me realize that my life had meaning, that I brought happiness to the most important guy in my life—my dad.

In his last years, my dad lived at a veteran's hospital. The nurses took good care of him and my mom made countless trips to assure him that he was still loved by his bride. Unfortunately, it was during these last years of Dad's life that I was going through a very difficult time of my own. I was a single mom with two little girls. I worked a second shift, twelve hours a day, seven days a week, and found it hard to find the time and energy to make the long trip to see him as much as I would have liked. When I did go, I'd do as my mother did and pack a couple of cans of Pepsi on ice—but I also took something else.

Two remarkable things would happen when I visited my father during these times. The first was that when he saw me walk into the room, his face would light up with a smile that told me he knew who had just walked in. He couldn't say my name or one sentence that made any sense, but there was no doubt that he knew I was his Ticket. Those smiles made me feel like his little girl again, even though I was almost thirty years old.

The other remarkable thing began one day when the nurse showed me a photo of a pumpkin my dad had drawn. My dad had been an incredible artist in his life, and despite the fact that Alzheimer's had rendered him severely cognitively impaired, something incredible happened when you put a pencil in his hand: He still remembered how to draw with details, shading, and accurate perspective. After that, I would often bring a sketchpad and charcoal; a couple times, I was lucky enough to get him to do some drawing. During those times I think we both experienced some much-needed peace in our lives.

When those we love face the challenges of Alzheimer's so much is stripped away from their lives... and ours, too. Memories are gone, as is the ability to do so many of the things that brought us joy. My father showed me that it's possible for those with Alzheimer's to experience some of what they love. Those things may often lie dormant within their hearts and minds, but if we're lucky enough, they can break through and bring immeasurable joy. A smile of recognition. A picture of a pumpkin. Two things I had often taken for granted years before had now become priceless gifts passed from father to daughter.

For most of my life my dad told me that I was his "Ticket to Happiness," but when I look back and think about all the incredible moments I had with my dad, even moments where the throes of Alzheimer's could have shrouded my life in sorrow, it was he who was my Ticket to Happiness—and that happiness still fills my heart today.

~Amy L. Sayers

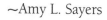

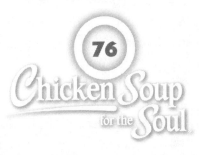

76

The Man in My Mother's Room

The desk has been shoved into a corner, its chair removed. The regular bed no longer reigns in the middle of the room, but has been reduced to a less important position closer to the window, a hospital bed serving as its companion. A recliner with giant arms competes for space. This piece, designed half as a sleeper and half as an ejector seat to help propel its occupant forward, is covered with sheets and a blanket.

The recliner plays a central role in the new dynamic here, alerting visitors to the troubles within these walls.

My mom is resting in it as I enter the room. Her eyes are closed, and she seems neither awake nor quite asleep. It is a condition that has become all too familiar. This room, this state of half being, is the place she inhabits with increasing frequency.

"Madam, your son Rob is here." My mom half opens her eyes.

"Rob?"

"Robert. I'm right here, Mom." I put my hand in hers and squeeze. She is surprisingly warm, and she squeezes back with a strength that acknowledges not only my presence, but also the depth of her feelings for me.

I try to talk with her, to keep her awake. It is only 5 p.m., but this has become her new bedtime. She has exchanged night for day, and sleep now comes at all the wrong hours. One of my roles is to keep her up just a bit longer, as we try to reset her clock, little by little.

I chronicle my day, and then a few seconds later I do it again. I make the smallest of small talk, trying anything that will keep her mind occupied. It is often a losing battle, and she drifts away.

In the background, there is the unmistakable voice of the 1940s. The boy from Hoboken is crooning in those gentle soothing tones, telling stories of love and tenderness. Suddenly, my mom raises an arm, acting as conductor to the band accompanying Sinatra. Then she begins to sing, in a clear voice. She recalls perfectly each syllable, each note. After several minutes, she grows quiet.

"Mom, did you ever see Sinatra perform?"

"Oh yes," she says. She is now more fully awake.

"It was really quite a few years ago." For a person who has lost any concept of her age, or where events occurred on a time line, this is an aberration.

"Do you remember who went with you to hear him? Where was it?" I know when her eyes move up and to the corner that she is searching her memory bank for clues. She tries to recall specifics but they're gone.

She begins to sing again, and I accompany her. I remember some of the words from the days I stood next to my dad, at the piano, reading over his shoulder as he played Sinatra in our living room. I squeeze my mom's hand to tell her how nice this is, and she reciprocates.

In a bit, she is silent. But I can sense how much she is enjoying the music. She conducts again in perfect rhythm. I stop trying to intercede and just let her have this time to herself, with Frank.

There is a man in my mom's bedroom, filling her mind and giving her comfort. She and Sinatra are in harmony. She is happy. And so am I.

~Robert S. Nussbaum

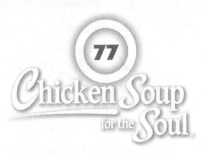

77

Herbert

A mother is a mother from the moment her baby is first placed in her arms until eternity.

~Sarah Strohmeyer

Mama's last child, Herbert, came into her life when she was eighty-seven. He was a rosy-cheeked fellow with one tiny white tooth. Dressed in newborn-size baby clothes and a pair of white shoes with my mother's name written in black marker on the soles, he tricked several people into believing he was real. Herbert was just a doll, but to my mama, he was a real child, and he became part of our family.

Mama acquired Herbert when she was in the late stage of Alzheimer's, a time when it was almost impossible for her to tell us what she felt, thought, needed, or wanted. But we learned, in this stage, just how deep her maternal instincts ran. She had devoted sixty of her eighty-eight years to caring for children or grandchildren, and she was warm, loving, and devoted. Holding a child in her arms was as natural to her as breathing, and being a good mother and grandmother was her mission in life. She was happiest when she was doing something for children, as she lovingly sacrificed her time, energy, and resources to make them happy—baking favorite desserts, helping with homework, having tea parties, wrestling with action figures, and playing board games.

And we, her children, desperately wanted to save her from the devastation of Alzheimer's. The disease forced us to reverse roles as she gradually lost the ability to understand and react to the world. Bit by bit, over eight years, she lost herself—memory, reading, writing, talking, the ability to care for herself, and ultimately, the ability to swallow. She was now the one who needed help, eventually moving into a nursing home where she could have the necessary supervision and professional care.

We tried to salvage any peace or pleasure we could in her new environment. When her mental capacity reached end stage but her physical body remained strong, she was trapped in a strange, dangerous, lonely world we could reach on only rare occasions. Hearing of the comfort that doll therapy can sometimes bring to people with Alzheimer's, we bought the lifelike doll that came to be known as Herbert.

We quickly learned that in Mama's eyes Herbert was real. Alzheimer's had long since robbed her of coherent conversation. But to our amazement, shortly after we gave her Herbert, she not only found the tune but also the words of a hymn to lull her baby to sleep as she rocked him in her arms. She still knew how to be a devoted caregiver.

Through her gestures and facial expressions, we learned Herbert was to be handled correctly, fed, admired, and loved. Shortly after Herbert came into her life, my brother was visiting, and needed to move Herbert, so he picked him up by the leg and dropped him in another spot. Her horror was apparent, and I suspect if she had had the capacity to call social services, we might have had some explaining to do. She also wanted to share her meals with Herbert. At mealtime, she would motion for us to spoon some of the food in Herbert's mouth as well. She was immensely proud of him.

I admit, at age fifty-seven, it felt a bit strange to be jealous of a doll. Herbert was her child, and I was… what? It was hard to determine if she knew me as anyone other than someone who came to visit. She would often focus her attention on Herbert rather than her "real" children who were trying to interact with her. She would point at him as she beamed proudly at his cute antics. She held and snuggled and cared; Herbert gave her back her greatest mission in life. She may have lost coherent words but not her ability to love her children.

Herbert was with her 24/7 and could accompany her to places we could not. When she fell or was sick and had to ride in the ambulance to the hospital, he went with her. Herbert had X-rays and MRIs along with her, and some of the hospital staff even came to know his name. We ensured that Herbert was by her side each time we left.

Eventually, the day arrived when not even Herbert could reach into Mama's world. A few days later, once again, he went with her as he rode to the funeral home snuggled in her arms. The next time we saw him, he was in her casket.

How I wish I could tell Mama how very proud I am of her. With Herbert's help, she showed the world that nothing — not even Alzheimer's — was stronger than her love for her children.

~Dale Adams O'Neill

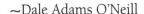

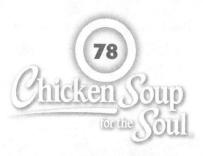

78

I Can't Help Falling in Love with You

To watch us dance is to hear our hearts speak.
~Hopi Indian Saying

At sixty-one my father was diagnosed with younger-onset Alzheimer's disease. The hints were subtle at first. He missed cues in conversation and told the same stories over and over again, but when my active, social father started avoiding family and talking all together, we knew something was wrong. Later, after many doctor's visits and failed attempts at drawing the face of a clock, we accepted the reality.

Eventually, my mom made the painful decision to move Dad into a nursing home. By that time, he needed help getting in and out of bed, going to the bathroom, even eating and walking. Soon I realized the nursing home was the best place for him. He couldn't wander off or be a threat to his own safety.

One day, Mom told me an Elvis impersonator was coming to the nursing home. I had never seen Elvis anywhere but on TV, so I didn't turn down the chance for a live performance. When Elvis finally came, a bit late, he arrived to the same game show-type soundtrack that accompanied the real Elvis. Don't think for a second he took it down a notch because of his surroundings; on the contrary, I think our Elvis was just as into the performance, if not more so, because he understood this would be the highlight of his audience's day. He was a one-man show, changing his music by himself and stepping out to the hallway once or twice for a costume change.

I was thoroughly enjoying myself, as were most people in the room. Dad was all smiles, and Mom laughed and tapped her foot, sometimes singing along, and grinning at Dad whenever he looked her way.

The audience sat in folding chairs along the side of the room, and I was sitting behind my parents. The center of the room was left open for our performer, and anyone who wanted to could come out and dance, or spin their wheelchairs in a circle.

When "I Can't Help Falling in Love with You" began to play, I had a feeling this was his last number: a nice slow song to close the show, calm everyone down, and send them off to their rooms. My dad turned his head to look at my mom, and the King came over to help him up so he could take my mom's hand and dance with her.

I was so happy for them and so sad at the same time. I didn't know if the tears welling up in my eyes were from joy or sorrow. But now I know. In front of me were two people who loved each other so much that even a debilitating, ruthless disease couldn't make them forget how important they were to one another, dancing right there in the middle of the tiled floor of the all-purpose room.

It didn't matter that the song was sung by an Elvis impersonator; it didn't matter that they were surrounded by other sick people and the staff who cared for them; it didn't even matter that Dad wouldn't remember this dance thirty minutes from now. What mattered was that they were together. "Take my hand. Take my whole life too. For I can't help falling in love with you."

Elvis, a veteran performer, could see my parents were a couple, and that I was their daughter. When his finale ended, and I was still trying to hide my watery eyes and blotchy complexion, he came over and handed me his scarf.

"I bet it's good to see them like that again," he said. "I'm guessing you haven't seen it in a while." I nodded, as a fresh batch of tears welled up in my eyes. The King squeezed my shoulder, and then Elvis left the building.

~Laurie Rueter Schultz

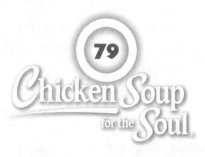

79

Hidden Talents

Any human anywhere will blossom in a hundred unexpected talents and
capacities simply by being given the opportunity to do so.
~Doris Lessing

t is still hard to believe, but my family and I only discovered my father's amazing artistic talent after he was diagnosed with Alzheimer's disease. Before age eighty-nine, he had no interest in painting a room, let alone a landscape.

Five years after his diagnosis, Dad began attending an Alzheimer's-based community day care center. During a painting class, the facilitator played music and used an Alzheimer's Association Memories in the Making art program to stimulate Dad's thought process. In no time, my father picked up a paintbrush for the first time and created his own form of artistic poetry.

Those who have seen my father's pictures can hardly believe them. The paintings are beautifully composed, colorful, and evoke memories of my grandmother and mother's flower gardens. My sisters and I now know where we get our artistic tendencies—before, we had no clue.

With support and encouragement from friends, my family and I are working to preserve my father's artistic legacy and help others living with Alzheimer's. We created notecards featuring four of his paintings and offer them at Alzheimer's-related events all around the state. Our family has raised thousands of dollars for the Alzheimer's Association Southeastern Virginia Chapter.

An unexpected yet gratifying outcome of my father's diagnosis has been my involvement in the Memories in the Making art program. I am now a trained facilitator who travels to memory care facilities to help residents create amazing pieces of art. The stories they share while painting, and their sense of accomplishment, give me so much satisfaction. I know my father would be proud of me. Without him, none of this would have happened.

My family and I are not only raising donations and awareness for Alzheimer's disease, but we are also looking to provide hope to caregivers and family members of those affected. The message is a powerful one: There may be another dimension to their loved ones that has yet to be discovered!

~Marjorie Hilkert

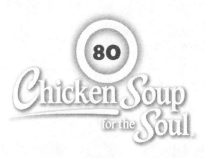

Music Therapy

Music is the universal language of mankind.
~Henry Wadsworth Longfellow

ivil War-era lawyer, orator, and social activist Robert
Ingersoll said, "Music expresses feeling and thought,
without language; it was below and before speech, and it
is above and beyond all words." Ingersoll's words resonate
with me, for Alzheimer's disease has snatched ordinary words from
my father. He now speaks solely in Italian, reverting to the language
of his youth—an even crueler change for a deeply intellectual man
who once knew several languages as a humanities professor. Although
I attempt Italian, my grammar is so broken that no deep thoughts are
possible, only fractured phrases conveying trivial facts, such as the
year I graduated from college. Even if I were to perfect this language,
there would still be a disconnect because he uses the Sardo dialect, a
tongue virtually impossible to those outside of the island.

Instead, I communicate with my father through the piano. The
scene is always the same: My mother and I push my father's wheelchair through the halls of the nursing home and place him at the perfect distance from the massive mahogany instrument. My mother's
friends shuffle in as well, pushing their loved ones into the lobby and
chattering about whether I will play "Take Me Out to the Ball Game"
because of the afternoon's baseball game.

I sit at the padded bench, my fingers tingling. As my hands
assume a life of their own, I summon the love I cannot verbally

express and project it through the black and white keys. The first song I play for him is Franz Schubert's "Ave Maria." After such a serious opening act, I try to liven the mood with "When the Saints Go Marching In," "You Are My Sunshine," and "Oh! Susanna." (I'll never understand why a man who grew up in Europe finds solace in this Southern anthem.)

After I finish, I breathlessly wait for his response "Stai molto bene!"

It is in his response that I feel fulfilled, because I realize we are still able to connect despite the clutches of this leech that is slowly sucking the life from my father. When I see how my father's face and the faces of dozens who gather to participate in this Sunday ritual light up, I think that an even higher level of cognitive functioning happens. I believe that the music transcends ordinary boundaries and expresses the intangible, a heightened form of expression not possible with words alone.

Because it stems from our souls and pours into our hearts, no translator misinterprets the message. Undoubtedly, music alone is the universal language.

~Kristina Aste-Mayer

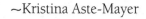

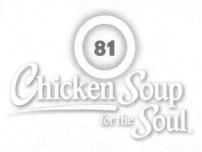

Holding On to Dad Through Alzheimer's

The value of identity of course is that so often with it comes purpose.
~Richard Grant

lzheimer's wasn't an unknown disease in our family. My grandmother was the first person I knew who had Alzheimer's; she passed away when I was nine. After Grandma it was Uncle John, followed by Aunt Shirley, and then Uncle Har, who is still living with the disease.

When my dad was diagnosed I thought the family was as prepared as we could be. I also believed my dad was prepared and accepted the diagnosis well. It wasn't until the second doctor's appointment that I realized he didn't take the news well at all. Mom, Dad, and I sat in the doctor's office as the doctor told us what to expect and discussed possible medications for managing symptoms.

We walked out of the office and Dad stopped in the hallway and stood for a moment. I asked if he was all right. Dad said, "I guess I didn't really believe the first doctor, but now two doctors agree. I guess I really have this disease."

The man who I always looked to when I needed support broke into tears and went limp in my arms. I just hugged him and supported him as much as I could.

I knew this disease and I knew it was a race against time, as his memories would slip away with every tick of the clock. Dad had a very aggressive form and seemed to go through the stages within weeks when other relatives had taken years. I spent most nights in tears but also reading, not about potential cures, but how I could help Dad with basic day-to-day activities.

One night I read something that changed my life. It was a comment on a blog suggesting that someone with Alzheimer's might not remember family members but might recognize simple relationships such as the nurse who brings them their favorite pudding. That night I started thinking about something I could do with Dad, like a hobby, which would differ from our father-daughter relationship. Dad was in great physical health and he had been a member of our local gym. I decided we would go to the gym together every Monday, Wednesday, and Friday. This fit with other articles that I read, which suggested that physical activity might help people with Alzheimer's disease.

We started going to the gym. In the beginning he remembered me, but as the months passed he would start to forget me on and off. I tried not to push him, and usually just answered his questions until he figured out who I was or what our relationship was. One beautiful warm day we decided to skip the gym and take a walk around his neighborhood. As we walked he told me about the people who lived in each house and which houses had dogs.

"Do you live around here?" Dad asked me.

"No, I live about five miles north. But I grew up in this neighborhood."

"Oh, do you know my son, Ken?"

"Yes, we played together a lot when we were young."

"Oh my gosh, you're my daughter, aren't you?" Dad asked with a huge smile on his face as if he had just found an old friend.

"Yes, I am," I said, turning my face away trying to hide my tears.

My idea worked. As Dad remembered our relationship less and less he still recognized me as a friend. Our relationship took a few unexpected turns during our days together but they were always positive. What I became in his mind was a taxi driver, friend, and fitness instructor.

I realized I was a taxi driver on our way to the gym once when Dad asked about my fees.

"How do you know how many miles you're driving me? You don't have a meter or anything. Shouldn't you have a meter so you know how much to charge people?"

"I drive to the gym all the time so I know how far it is; it doesn't change." I answered his questions as I always did, without pushing him to remember me.

"How many people do you drive like me?"

"Just you," I said as we pulled onto the highway.

"Well, you can't make much money doing that. I don't go out much."

"It's okay; I have other sources of income. Don't worry about me." This sounded like the dad I knew, always worried about having an income and health insurance.

"Well, who pays you to drive me around?"

"Nobody. I don't get paid." Sometimes my mom gave me gas money, but I didn't want to explain that so I stuck with the simple answer.

"Why do you do this, I mean drive me around?" Dad asked, still trying to figure out who I was and why I would spend time with him.

"Because I love you," I said, still looking straight ahead.

"Oh, isn't that nice." And that seemed to satisfy his curiosity for the day.

On another occasion Dad almost fired me. We took our regular walk around the track at the gym. As we walked Dad began to ask questions about my training and certification to work as a fitness instructor.

"How did you learn to do this?" Dad asked.

"What do you mean?"

"Well, help me and these other people with our fitness programs. Did you go to school for fitness?"

"No, I'm not a trainer, I just come here and walk with you," I said as we continued to walk.

"You mean you're not certified to help me? How do you know I'm doing the right program?"

"I don't. We're just walking and stuff," I said, not knowing how to respond without scaring him.

Dad was silent for a few minutes and that's when I figured he was thinking about firing me. How would that look on a résumé?

"So, do you have any education or certification for anything?" Dad finally said.

"I have a master's degree in Business Administration, an MBA," I said.

"Oh, well, I guess with that you can probably do just about any job you want," Dad said with a little chuckle.

Getting my degree was an important moment in my life. It meant a lot to me to know that even though Dad didn't remember me, he was still impressed by my accomplishment.

A few weeks before we lost Dad, he told me that he didn't always remember me as his daughter but he always knew he could trust me and that he was safe with me.

Help them feel safe. That's the best advice I can give to a care-giver of someone with Alzheimer's disease. It worked for me, and it gave me a continuing relationship with my father right till the end.

~Julie Staffen

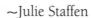

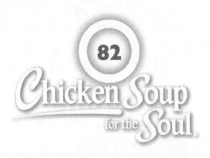

The Pianist

All deep things are song. It seems somehow the very central essence of us,
song; as if all the rest were but wrappages and hulls!
~Thomas Carlyle

The floors of the old church creaked and popped as we maneuvered the antique piano across the scarred floorboards. The piano was an ornate upright, a remnant of the days when piano keys were made of ebony and ivory. I'm certain it outweighed a Volkswagen Beetle. It was a treasured donation to an old country church built in the 1870s, which had just undergone a restoration after a half-century of neglect and storm damage. I couldn't wait for music to fill the sanctuary again.

My aunt, Alison, and her husband, Don, had recently arrived from Ohio for their annual visit, each thousand-mile trip made incrementally more difficult by Don's advancing Alzheimer's. Although he had medication to manage the disease symptoms, the changes wrought by the passage of each year were painful to watch. As half a dozen of us carefully moved the piano across the floor, rolling it over pieces of thick plywood to avoid putting too much weight on one floorboard, Don stood silently at the back of the church and watched.

A scientist with a doctorate in polymer chemistry, Don was slender, with a full head of white hair rivaling Toscanini's mane. His illness had gradually robbed him of the ability to make conversation. He kept a small notebook in his shirt pocket on which he noted the date and day of the week. Sometime during the past year all names had deserted him, except for Alison's. She was his anchor, and he kept her in sight as much as possible, becoming uneasy when she made trips to the bathroom. My heart went out to her in her state of constant vigilance. Yesterday we had found him outside searching through the wrong car for his jacket.

The call for help to move the piano had resulted in the gathering of a small crowd, many of whom made polite attempts to initiate conversation with Don. But his repertoire of stories had diminished and the conversations didn't last long. He wandered outside under the shade of the live oaks, but returned often to mark the slow progress of the piano and our attempts to center it on a sheet of plywood in the front corner of the church.

Music stitched together Don's family. He and each of his four children played instruments with professional expertise: piano, violin, viola, flute. They sang in their church choir. I'll never forget his look of pained horror when we celebrated the birthday of one of our grandchildren a few years back with a rousing chorus of "Happy Birthday." We are a large, multigenerational family and sang hopelessly off-key, our tempo far too slow. Don made us start over while he conducted.

When the piano was finally installed, we adjourned to a shady spot under the trees and broke open a cooler of sodas. A homecoming celebration was in the works, with invitations going out to all who had ties to the old church during its long history as the center of a tiny Texas community. As we discussed plans for the event, music began to waft from the open windows. Mozart. Heads turned and conversations halted. Even the birds stopped singing. "Who's playing that?" someone asked. It was Don.

I know that people with Alzheimer's lose recent memories first while retaining memories from the distant past. Don's early piano studies were firmly entrenched. He had no sheet music; the complex sonata was still fixed in a part of his brain not yet damaged by the disease.

We drifted silently into the back of the church, doing our best not to disturb him, but he had closed his eyes and was lost in the music.

"How do you do that?" my brother asked when Don got up from the piano stool.

"It's what I've always done," he said.

It has been nearly three years since that day, and Don has since moved into an Alzheimer's facility that can provide the specialized care he needs. He still plays the piano in the recreation room to the delight of other patients. And whenever I slide the dust cover off that old church piano, I think of the day he proved to all of us that amid the fog of Alzheimer's, the light of music was still shining.

~Martha Deeringer

Seek support and stay connected.
It is important to stay engaged in
meaningful relationships and
activities. Whether family,
friends or a support group, a
network is critical.

"Five steps to overcome Alzheimer's stigma"
alz.org/ihavealz

Living
with Alzheimer's
& Other Dementias

It Takes a Village

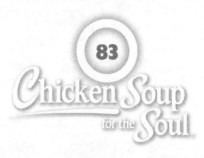

We're All Family Here

The charity that is a trifle to us can be precious to others.
~Homer, The Odyssey

My father spent the last three years of his life in the secured ward of a memory care unit. In December 2011, he lost the ability to swallow and my family and I cared for him during his final days. But this story isn't about my dad's departure; it's about those he left behind on the second floor, and two men who have convinced me that angels come in the strangest shapes and sizes.

My brothers, Russ and Reed, are both in their sixties. They have worked for decades in a family business that requires physical strength, creative thinking, and people skills. They are hunters and fishermen; they love bicycles and motorcycles, an occasional cigar, and Maker's Mark. They revered my dad and visited him often. In fact, the director of the memory care unit, which typically cares for about twenty-five residents, told us that our family paid more visits to my father than all of the other residents' families combined.

But my brothers went far, far beyond the call of duty. Over time they got to know virtually everyone on the second floor—staff members and residents alike. During my father's last week, I got to know many of them through my brothers' eyes.

"That's Dora," Russ said, pointing to a petite Latino woman. "She's from Managua and used to own several beauty salons. Very astute businesswoman in her day."

Dora looked around with a puzzled expression. "Why am I here?" she asked.

My brother shook his head. "The fact that she asks the question answers her question, don't you think?"

A slender, dapper gentleman sat at a table. Kenny was a Royal Air Force mechanic. He grew up in Portsmouth, England, and his family owned a toy store. Often he would relive his World War II experience.

"At the rat tat tat tat tat we would have to scurry into the trenches to avoid being injured," he recounted in his proper British accent.

At other times Kenny asked Russ if he'd seen his wife.

"No I haven't," Russ always said. "But if I see her I'll let her know you're looking for her." Kenny's wife had been dead since 1994.

Peter came prancing by. He was German and full of energy. He loved to sing and dance. He carried a flashlight wherever he went, and on this occasion he was worried because it wasn't working. My brother Reed promised Peter he'd bring him batteries next time — and he did.

Peter was in the German army, and one day Russ sat him down with my dad, whose liberty ship was sunk by a German U-boat in the Atlantic in 1945. "Peter, your country's navy sunk my dad's ship in the war."

"Oh, I'm sorry about that," Peter replied, contrite.

My father waved his hand. "All is forgiven." And in the world of the second floor, where the most reliable memories are more than half a century old, that said a lot.

I was walking down the hall with Reed and a head popped out of a room — at floor level. It was Monroe, a P-51 mechanic in World War II and now a Dallas Cowboys fan. He forgets he can't walk and often slips out of his wheelchair. I panicked, ready to call for help.

"Hello Monroe," Reed greeted him, helping him back into his chair before continuing down the hall. "Happens all the time," he told me. "No biggie."

During that final week I spent a lot of time on the second floor. My brothers, their wives, my mother, and other family members would come and go. At lunchtime someone would run out for sandwiches; we'd eat them in a small common room at the end of the hall. Sometimes Wanda would join us. Once a sergeant in the Air Force, Wanda was friendly, engaging and seemed quite "with it," except that she remembered very little about herself. Still, she was welcome to share our meal and often did.

One evening as we sat with my dad, a resident named Donna, who was wheelchair-bound, rolled into the room. Normally very loving and clear-eyed, she was obviously upset.

"What's wrong, Donna?" Russ asked, putting his arm around her. "Are you lost?"

She nodded tearfully.

"I'll take you back where you belong," he said. "Don't worry." The compassion in my brother's voice made me want to weep.

Over several days my dad grew weaker. "He is actively dying," the hospice workers told us. On one of his last nights, Toni wandered into the room. She was wraithlike, much too slender, with long gray hair; dementia had her securely in its clutches. She would often take Russ's face in her hands and say "Panos? Panos?" which was the name of her son. My brother would nod and she would coo lovingly to him in Greek.

Russ tells the story of one day when he noticed Toni walking with a man who could be her son. "Are you Panos?" my brother asked him.

The man looked surprised. "Yes, I am."

"So am I," Russ said with a grin. The man began to apologize for his mother, but my brother stopped him.

"We're in this together," Russ said. "We're all family here."

When Toni wandered in that evening, the atmosphere was subdued. We were playing one of Dad's favorite CDs softly and the lights were low. We were all somber because we knew our vigil was coming to an end. Toni said nothing, but looked at all of us and gave the sign of the cross. And just as quietly she left.

The next evening my father died. Many of the staff members cried, but Rolando, the maintenance man, was serene. Days before, at my brothers' request, he had given my dad a blessing. They have been around Rolando long enough to believe he's a holy man.

"You do not need to worry," Rolando told me. "Your papa is in good hands."

Alzheimer's is an insidious disease that stealthily robs us of what we value most: our sense of who we are. But to the end, every person with dementia remains a person with a story—an individual who worked, and loved, and lived a worthwhile life. The number of people with Alzheimer's is growing, and we need more "angels" like my brothers, individuals who are willing to say to people who will never truly know them, "You matter to me, even now."

The funny part is, Russ and Reed will tell you angels have nothing to do with it. "They're my friends," Russ would say. And Reed would just roll his eyes, as if to say, "What's the big deal?"

My dad is gone and there's no reason for my brothers to visit the second floor anymore. But they do. The other day Russ met a new woman, Aileen. She had an accent and he asked her where she was from.

"France," she replied. "Bordeaux."

"Ah," my brother said. "Wine-making country."

"Oui," she said, her eyes lighting up. "Delicious wines."

"So, Aileen, will you be my friend?" Russ asked.

"Oui, Certainement," she said.

It's as easy—and as awe-inspiring—as that.

~Louise Harris Berlin

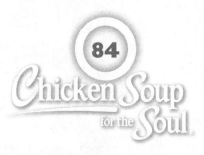

84

My Valentine

Oh, if it be to choose and call thee mine, love,
thou art every day my Valentine!
~Thomas Hood

Valentine's Day has always been a big deal at our house. Although my husband is a year-round romantic, John feels that this is the day to put the icing on the love cake.

Our celebrations have ranged from a quiet, candlelit dinner in a pricey French restaurant to a wild, pizza-fueled, weekend sleepover with our grandkids. No matter how we marked the occasion, Valentine's Day was always filled with love and gratitude for the life we created together. This year we decided to avoid the crowds and went out to dinner a few days early, but kept our tradition of not exchanging cards until "the day."

John elevated Valentine card shopping into a high art form. He could spend hours looking for the perfect sentiment. Mostly romantic, sometimes funny, his choices clearly reflected what was going on in our life at the time. He took this task so seriously that he kept the location of his favorite card store a secret. However, this year would be different. John was living with Alzheimer's disease, and because of his diagnosis, he could no longer drive.

As Valentine's Day drew near, John became anxious because he had not been able to go card shopping. I told him not to worry, that I would drive him to the store and he could pick something out. This bothered him even more. How could he find the perfect card if I was hovering in the background? And what about flowers? Where was he going to get the long-stemmed red roses that he wanted to give me?

My aunt came to our rescue by asking a simple question: "What can I do for you today?" We jumped at the opportunity for her to take John to the store. Unsure if John had enough money, I pressed some bills into her hand while he was getting ready to go. To her raised eyebrow I responded, "Tell him that is his budget." They bundled themselves into the car and off they went.

I didn't realize until that moment how important it was to the both of us to have another year of surprise. When I later mentioned this to a friend, she said she would put all of our important dates on her calendar and make sure to take him shopping each time.

I received a bouquet of beautiful red tulips and, as usual, his card was perfect. In essence it told me of his gratitude to me for listening, for lifting him when he stumbles, and for laughing with him. For being his one and only Valentine.

~Angie Carrillo

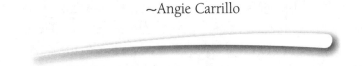

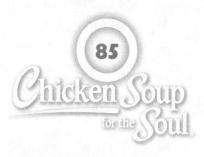

85

Still Sancho

I know who I am and who I may be, if I choose.
~Miguel de Cervantes, Don Quixote

"**D**id you make that?" a chirpy voice asked. I looked around and saw the Laundromat was deserted (or so I'd assumed). Then I saw her—a white-haired old lady. At four feet ten inches, she was a peanut.

She smiled, asking again, "Sorry, but I was just wondering if you made that," pointing to the granny square lap robe somersaulting in a nearby dryer. She added, "I used to crochet, years ago." We chatted, exchanging names. Kitty and I became instant friends.

The conversation went on. For more than a decade. We talked about food, love, religion—our unhappy childhoods. Once, I recall tittering like schoolgirls over a handsome young Spanish actor we slyly nicknamed "Tony Flags." It was the literal translation of his name. So what if everybody else called him Antonio Banderas?

Kitty is older than my birth mother, yet she and I always had the feeling ours was a bond between contemporaries. I have never been sure why. She had a curiosity about life, the sort more often found in much younger people. Maybe that was it. Truth is, we got on superbly. No generation gap.

My neighbor Barbara, seeing us walking one day, chuckled that we looked like Don Quixote and his faithful squire Sancho Panza, on a quest for a windmill in need of tilting. The nicknames stuck and defined my relationship with Kitty in the profoundest way. Often before we would head out adventuring, Kitty would ask if I had my keys and subway tokens.

Then I'd ask her if she had used the bathroom, or if her shoes would serve for the trek. The collar on my favorite denim shirt had a nasty habit of flipping up. She'd reach up, smooth it back down and say, "Now we're ready."

Kitty was an avid bookworm who loved detective stories and historical fiction. She read cookbooks as one might read a novel. A crossword buff, she waggishly boasted, "I prefer the term cruci-verbalist!"

As the years went on she started losing language. Slowly, subtly. A phrase here, a noun there. She would refer to something as a "whatchamacallit." I found this quirk annoying and chided Kitty for being lazy. It never occurred to me I was seeing early signs of an illness that would eventually bring the briskly turning gears of an exceptionally busy mind to a near halt. Some time later, during one of our daily phone chats, I asked what she was doing. "Cleaning," she quietly answered. "The... big white... thing in the kitchen. You put food in it?"

A short while later her facility with crossword puzzles abruptly disappeared. Almost as if some phantom eraser had swooped down and begun, bit by bit, rubbing things out of her brain. Kitty's relatives moved her to a nursing home six months later.

Trying to arm myself against the inevitable, I read whatever I could find about Alzheimer's. I learned that a person who has Alzheimer's can still experience the world through the senses: sight, sound, touch, smell. Thinking back on our years together, I would visit Kitty in the nursing home with some item or other in tow. Gazing into her blank face, I would place an object in her lap.

Her doctor, seeing me there one afternoon, stopped by to talk. She made a point to tell me, "Alzheimer's is by no means straight downhill, you know. Remember to expect surprises."

Then and there I decided to put my despair on hold as much as possible. I promised myself I would keep up what I had come to call The Bringing: a bracelet of dark wooden beads, scented with sandalwood. A handful of dried lavender bundled in a lace doily. Two braided macramé belts—one pink, the other deep purple. At the farmer's market, I bought broccoli florets, a favorite of ours when we cooked together in my phone booth-sized kitchen. Smooth black stones from a neighbor's bonsai garden. My hope, of course, was to awaken her from her stupor, if only for a moment. And indeed, she would sometimes take one of the objects in her hand, sparking briefly. Then the fog would settle in once more.

Since by this time she could no longer walk, I needed a way to get physically near to her in her bulky wheelchair. I moved closer, pressed my forehead against hers. Looking for a way to break through to my old pal, my Sancho Panza, I asked myself, "Perhaps a song will do?" Kitty loved "You Are My Sunshine." I looked out the window, noticed it was raining. No sunshine here, I thought. Pulling the folding metal chair nearer I leaned in, took a breath, and sang the first lines in her ear.

Her eyes were closed, head bowed onto her chest. In almost a whisper I began, "You are my sunshine, my only sunshine, you make me happy, when skies are gray." Within seconds Kitty lifted her head, joined her voice to mine, word for word, note for note in exactly the same key. We sang it together twice through. Only by then, I was the one having trouble.

She turned to face me. During the song I hadn't noticed—the shirt I had on was that old worn denim one. The collar had turned the wrong way. With the same loving, gentle precision I remembered from years ago, Sancho's hand reached up. And put it right.

~Cindy Legorreta

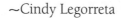

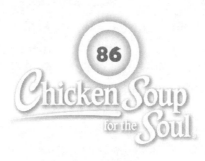

TGIF

There is no psychiatrist in the world like a puppy licking your face.
~Ben Williams

The door opens and the woman who peers out at me looks somewhat apprehensive, leaving the door only slightly cracked. "Yes?" she asks softly.

Then she looks down, and when she sees my two Shih Tzus wagging their tails, her face lights up. She opens the door wide, her arms out to welcome us in.

"Oh, I hoped it would be you!" she says excitedly, clapping her hands together. She calls out to her husband, who is napping but wakes up as soon as he hears his name.

"Fred! Look who it is! It's Panda and Koala!" Then she turns to me with a sheepish grin. "And Geoff and Kristi too, of course."

She walks over and wraps my husband in a loving embrace. "I'm so glad you came."

She talks as she shuffles along in front of us. "You know, I've been thinking about you all week. On Wednesday I wondered if you were coming and yet you didn't. Then yesterday I thought we'd missed you, but then I told myself, no Helen, Friday. That's the day they come. And now, here it is!"

I smile at her enthusiasm. I encourage them to make themselves comfortable in their recliners and then carefully put one dog on each of their laps. They sit patiently while I pull bags of dog treats out of my pocket. Then they spend the next several minutes trying to get their stiff, arthritic fingers into the bags to dig out the treats for Panda and Koala.

"Your cough is gone." Helen says to Geoff. "You look much better today." My heart fills. Not only did she remember him, she remembered that he'd been sick.

Helen and Fred are just some of the residents in the Alzheimer's unit we visit once a week. I've been bringing my dogs here for nine months now. My husband joined me recently and has become almost as attached to the routine as I have.

I watch Helen stroking Koala until he lies on his side and closes his eyes. I marvel at how easy it has become for her to get my formerly abused and shy little dog to relax completely. She will stroke and talk softly to him for most of our visit.

"They are just the sweetest things," she whispers.

Panda is sprawled across Fred's lap. He's rubbing her belly and her eyes begin to close in contentment.

"Oh, I just love these two little buggers," Fred says chuckling.

He points at the framed collage I made for them with pictures of each dog, the two of them together and the four of us, all with labels in big lettering.

"Do you know that's one of my favorite things? Now let's see, this one here," he points to Panda, "Is the one in the top right picture?"

"Yep," I say. "The one labeled Panda."

"Yes, Fred. You can tell by the white spot on the head. See?" Helen points to the smaller spot on Koala's head. "This is the one in the top left. Right?" she looks at me questioningly.

"Right!" I say, smiling. I noticed she remembered the white spot reference I'd provided several visits ago.

Geoff begins to talk about his work with fish and wildlife.

"That's what I did, you know," Fred says.

"I know," Geoff says. "Tell me the deer-in-the-cage story again."

Fred chuckles and tells us the story. We laugh and ask the right questions. And occasionally Helen adds something. Or she turns to me and points to Koala and giggles. She can't remember where they lived or her sons' ages, but she remembers that Koala snores.

It's never easy to end the visits. But at some point we have to and Fred and Helen reluctantly bid goodbye to Panda and Koala. They give us each a hug.

"You take care of yourself," Fred tells us.

"We'll see you next Friday, okay?" we tell them, stressing the word *Friday*.

Then we head into the lounge. Despite saying goodbye to them in their room, Fred and Helen have followed us out.

"Be careful with those mean dogs," Fred says, laughing. Helen giggles.

We make our way out, stopping for the staff members who kneel down to get kisses and sneezes from the dogs. No matter how long we're there, I'm constantly astounded by the effect the dogs have on the residents. They remember us, they remember the dogs, and it brings out memories, stories, and songs. It calms them and makes them visibly happy.

It's not easy to become attached to someone and then lose them, but we do it because it makes our day as much as it does theirs. So many of them tell us how much they miss their own dogs. Sharing ours for a couple hours is the least we can do.

I wave to Fred and Helen as we go.

"You're just the best part of my week," she says, and my heart is full.

~Kristi Cocchiarella FitzGerald

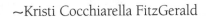

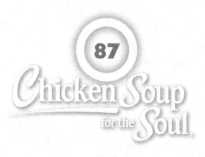

A Plate of Cookies

Cookies are made of butter and love.
~Norwegian Proverb

t was Christmas Eve and I had just finished putting the last of the glaze and sprinkles on a batch of Christmas cookies. I remembered how my mother and I used to spend the holidays mixing the ingredients, cutting out the shapes and meticulously decorating each one. We would put so much love and time into those cookies every year, and then pass them out to friends and family members. I learned from my mother that we weren't just making cookies, but gifts of the heart.

This all changed when my mother got Alzheimer's disease. I still made cookies, but she wasn't by my side adding her touch.

My mother's younger brother Wayne also had Alzheimer's. He had just moved into a new care home and because it was Christmas Eve I went to visit him with a plate of those beloved holiday treats. He seemed happy to see my cousin and me, and we settled ourselves on the couch next to his wheelchair to talk about the day.

"What do you have there?" he asked, pointing to my plate.

"I have Christmas cookies. Would you like one? I know it isn't Christmas without a plate of my mother's cookies!"

"Sure," he said. I took off the plastic wrap and handed him one.

A few minutes later, he looked at me with a few crumbs on his face and said, "What do you have there?" pointing to my plate.

"I have Christmas cookies. Would you like one?"

"Sure," he said, and ate another cookie.

My uncle had a great twinkle in his eye and when he looked over again, I could see it.

"What do you have there?" he asked.

"Well, Uncle Wayne, I made Mom's Christmas cookies. Would you like one?"

"Sure," he said and reached for another.

My cousin and I chatted for a bit longer and within the next twenty minutes, Uncle Wayne asked the same question repeatedly, until there were only a couple of cookies left on the plate. It was getting late, so I kissed him goodbye, leaving him with the cookies and promising to return soon.

But I didn't get a chance to keep my promise, as he passed away just a few weeks later. I was heartbroken. At his funeral service, my cousin pulled me aside and told me the story of those last remaining cookies. Apparently, Uncle Wayne finished eating all but one of the cookies. He carried that last cookie with him everywhere. Every morning he would gently place the decorated cookie into his brown-plaid flannel shirt pocket and in the evening he would gently slip it out of his pocket and tuck it under his pillow.

What a comfort and a blessing to know the rest of the story. I know that he could feel the love that I mixed into those ingredients that day, and although the disease didn't allow him to let me know how he felt, his gestures and that twinkle in his eye did.

~W. Bond

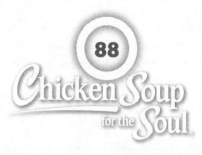

Unsung Heroes

*Unselfish and noble actions are the most radiant pages
in the biography of souls.*
~David Thomas

Mom was coming home, and I didn't know what to do. A surprise diagnosis of "normal pressure hydrocephalus" and a shunt insertion had brought an amazing turnaround. She had spent three months in a skilled nursing facility and another two weeks in grueling in-patient rehabilitation. Even after all that, she would be able to do very little on her own and was at high risk of falls. And we still had to contend with her dementia.

I needed help. But where would I find it? I researched in-home care agencies, but the cost nearly made me pass out. Surely we could find another way. I put out the word at church that I was looking for caregivers and called friends asking them to do the same at their churches. I took a chance on one unlikely source, a homeschool e-mail loop, where I sent a plea for help. Word spread.

It worked, and over the next three years, God brought some amazing women into our lives. Each had a unique personality and gifts that enriched both my mother's life and mine in ways I would never have imagined.

Cheri, with the spiked hair and beautiful smile, loved to do nails. She also loved to talk. Mom often felt she was left out of things because her hearing deteriorated shortly after surgery and she couldn't understand much of what we said. Cheri would get right down in Mom's face while filing and buffing her nails, and they would talk and talk. I always knew when Cheri had worked because Mom showed off her latest nail color and gave me the scoop on happenings in Cheri's neighborhood.

Charlotte, a widow, was tall, well spoken, and unflappable. She could calm Mom during her rages when the rest of us couldn't. Mom loved Charlotte because she treated her with quiet kindness, but Charlotte also possessed another priceless skill. She could do hair. Each time Mom's hair grew out after her shunt revisions, Charlotte colored it the ash blond Mom favored and gave her a perm. In between, she pin-curled and styled it. She would never take extra money for her work. These might have seemed like small things in Mom's overall care, but they were huge for her sense of wellbeing.

Then there was Joan, who came to work for us at the beginning and stayed until the end. A short powerhouse of a woman, Joan was practical and organized. I called her my right-hand woman. She instituted The Notebook, where caregivers could leave notes for each other on Mom's current preferences, complaints, and needs—what worked and what didn't. She asked me to print a chore list so they could coordinate keeping the house clean. Not that cleanliness was an issue when Joan was around. I often walked in to find her with her head stuck in the refrigerator scrubbing shelves or up on a stool straightening cabinets. She even tried to mow the yard during one of Mom's naps but couldn't get the mower started.

When Mom had a doctor's appointment, Joan often came in early to get her ready and to sweep or de-ice the wheelchair ramp. Upon my arrival, Joan would hand me a list of Mom's blood pressure readings neatly copied out for the cardiologist, or her food diary for the gastroenterologist. Many times she included Mom's lunchtime meds in a bag, "in case you run late or want to stop for lunch."

But Joan's caregiving went beyond practicality. On her days off or when she went on vacation, she called to check on Mom. She visited her during hospitalizations and brought gifts or cooked food she thought Mom would like. Joan showed she cared in a thousand ways, as did all our caregivers. And there were many. Some stayed a short time or came late in the course of Mom's illness, but they all showed unconditional love nonetheless.

And it wasn't always easy. As anyone who has cared for someone with dementia knows, the disease changes one's personality. My normally patient mother became demanding. She wanted things done now, if not sooner. Worst of all, Mom went through spells when she cursed the caregivers for the least infraction—or for none. There were days when no one could do anything right. More than once, I stopped by the house and found a caregiver in tears. Yet they stayed.

And more came.

Caryl was an excellent cook and baked mouthwatering pies to entice Mom to eat. She also knitted and made her a stylish scarf, a cup cozy, and a tissue holder. One night I visited and found Mom covered with the softest blanket I'd ever felt. She said Caryl had bought it to keep her extra warm.

Kristy came to work for us a few months before Mom passed away. A mother of four, she had a delightful sense of humor and the most gentle and nurturing nature. Toward the end, when Mom became irrationally fearful, Kristy would sit and hold her hand for hours. One chilly day, I walked in and found Kristy wearing a tank top and leaning over Mom. Her sweatshirt hung from one arm. My mother had grabbed Kristy's hand as she reached down to put fresh water on the table. When Kristy became unbearably warm, she pulled her sweatshirt over her head with her free hand rather than let go of Mom's hand.

Debbie worked with us on Sundays for several months. Even after her health problems required her to quit, she texted frequently to check in on Mom. The day before Mom passed away, Debbie showed up at the door. She wanted to see Mom one last time and sat holding her hand and praying for her.

How blessed we were by such compassionate women. They not only cared for Mom but also cared about her and became part of our family. These women may not have been classic heroes, but they rescued me when I needed them most. And though none were trained healthcare professionals, they were all exceptional caregivers.

~Tracy Crump

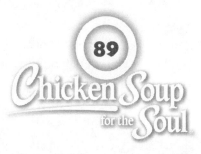

Those Damn Rings!

It is the greatest of all mistakes to do nothing
because you can only do little — do what you can.
~Sydney Smith

W hat was it about those damn rings? Why was she talking about them now? She hadn't worn her wedding
set for years, and now she was asking for it. Didn't she
remember that she was divorced? If we ever brought
up his name she got angry and left the room. She had taken those
rings off years ago and had not mentioned his name again. Didn't
she remember how much she disliked her ex-husband? I guess her
Alzheimer's had progressed enough to cleanse that memory.

My aunt could no longer live alone. She was unable to care for
herself and while she had moments of clarity, much of the time she
was living in the past and was confused. She had no children, so my
husband and I were in charge. We had to put her in an assisted living
facility for her own safety and for our peace of mind. That's when the
problem with the rings started.

At most assisted living facilities, residents cannot keep items of
value in their rooms. Money, credit cards and jewelry all fall in this
category. My aunt's wedding set was pretty flashy, with a big stone in
the middle of her engagement ring. There was no way Blanche, the
head of the facility, would allow her to wear her wedding set.

"Where are my damn rings?" she asked the day after we moved
her in.

"What rings?" I asked.

"You know damn well which rings I mean. I haven't taken my rings off for years, and now you are keeping them from me. Those rings are so very special to me. They were given to me by my devoted husband—the man I love. And now you won't give them to me. I want my rings. Now!"

I visited her almost every day, and every day instead of saying "Hello, nice to see you," she'd say, "Where are my damn rings and when are you going to give them back to me?"

I tried to focus her attention on something else. That didn't work. I tried substituting another ring for her wedding set but she would have none of that. She forgot so many things—what she had for lunch, that she had even had lunch. Why couldn't she forget about her rings? And why was I the bad guy? She never asked my husband where her rings were. She didn't get mad at him. Only me.

I tried to distract her but our conversations always came back to her rings. It became such a problem that I finally met with Blanche and talked to her about the situation. I told her that my aunt wanted her rings and nothing I did seemed to distract her from the subject. I told her I would sign a waiver stating that if anything happened to the rings I would not hold the facility liable. I would take full responsibility for the rings. Blanche was not happy about it, but she agreed that my aunt could have her rings back, because it would calm her and make her easier to deal with.

The next day, when I came to visit, I was greeted with the usual sour face and the question about her rings. I casually pulled them out of my pocket and handed them over. She was silent for the longest time and then she put them on. And then she smiled. At me! I told her that she needed to keep them safe and she should not take them off—ever. She assured me she would be careful.

The next time I visited she was pretty quiet and she had a towel over her hand. "What wrong with your hand?" I asked. "Nothing at all," she answered, and got up and closed the door. Then she looked left and right and whispered in a conspiratorial tone, "I'm hiding my rings so no one will see them."

"You don't have to do that, Aunt Clare. You wanted your rings, so you should wear them and enjoy them. People will think it's strange and wonder why you have a towel draped over your hand and it will draw even more attention to your rings."

When I got there the next day the rings were not on her hand. Oh no! I didn't know if she would remember where they were, but it didn't hurt to ask.

"Aunt Clare, I see that you're not wearing your rings. Where are they?"

She got this strange look on her face and once again got up and closed the door to her room. Then she looked left and right and came over to me and whispered, "I hid them."

Great! She had Alzheimer's and she had hidden her rings. Where in the world had she put them? Would she remember or were they lost forever? I had to try to find them so I whispered back, "Please show me where they are."

She thought for a long time and then slowly went over to her closet, opened the door, reached up on the shelf and there, wadded up in some tissue, were her rings. How easily those crumpled tissues could have been viewed as trash. This whole situation was going from bad to worse. It was almost funny, except it wasn't.

My poor aunt, who couldn't remember that she hated her ex-husband, did remember that I told her to be careful with her rings. Who knew what would happen the next time I came to visit? Where would the rings be?

When I arrived the next day she was sitting in the chair in her room looking out to the garden. I tried very hard not to look at her hand to see if she was wearing her rings. Don't look, I told myself... don't look... don't look. But I couldn't help myself. I looked, and there they were. On her finger. Safe.

But the look on her face told me she wanted to tell me something. I sat down and waited. Because of Alzheimer's, it usually took her a moment to organize her thoughts. She looked at me, looked at her rings, looked at me, and then back at her rings.

She took her rings off and handed them to me. "Here," she said.

"I don't think I should be wearing my rings in this place. I want you to have them; I'm done with them."

"Okay, Aunt Clare. I'll take them and I promise you I'll keep them safe." She smiled. I smiled. And she never spoke of her damn rings again!

~Madison Thomas

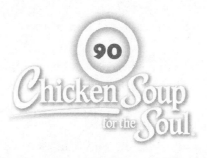

Remembering the Best Part

Love is a symbol of eternity. It wipes out all sense of time, destroying all memory of a beginning and all fear of an end.
~Author Unknown

I stopped at the desk to sign in and explained to the receptionist I was a reporter from the local newspaper and was doing a story on a gentleman who lived there, a World War II veteran. As I made my way down the corridor to Mr. Walter's room, I heard the receptionist behind me.

"Mrs. Dodson, you know Mr. Walter is practically deaf and suffers from dementia, don't you?"

"No ma'am, I didn't."

His daughter, who I'd spoken with days before, failed to mention his condition, but because I was already there I decided to go ahead with the interview.

As I passed room after room, each one looked the same: a single bed, a dark wooden nightstand, and a shiny brass lamp. I smiled at the elders sitting along the wall in their wheelchairs.

"Mr. Walter?" I read his name on the plaque outside his door, but I would have never recognized him by the picture his daughter had e-mailed the day before. A soldier dressed in army fatigues, tall and thin, but with broad shoulders and an even broader smile. It looked as if the photograph had captured him in the middle of a hilarious joke.

He looked up from a sunken blue chair, a blanket covering his lap. I could tell he didn't understand what I'd said. I sat down on the corner of his bed and introduced myself, stretching my hand out to his while he slowly shook it.

"Aw, you have soft skin!" he said hoarsely.

Luckily, he knew I was a reporter and that I'd come to interview him for a story on local veterans. We spoke for a few minutes, and although communicating was difficult because he was hard of hearing, he had a quick wit and made me feel at ease.

"Can you tell me a little about where you served in the army?" I asked.

The interview began like many others, I asked questions and he answered them. I'd learned over the years as a reporter to say as little as possible, allowing the person to do most of the talking. And Mr. Walter did.

He shared with me that he was a medic in World War II and during battles their battalion put crosses on their helmets signifying their position. Under the Geneva Convention, enemies weren't allowed to bomb his area.

"But it didn't always happen that way," Mr. Walter said.

I sat quietly, writing and listening, but in the middle of one of his recollections of the Battle of Normandy he blurted out, "And I drove so quick to JCPenney I nearly ran over a pedestrian!"

And so it went for thirty more minutes. Talks of soldiers and battle wounds mixed with Yankees baseball and his daughter's first communion.

Soon I put my notebook down and resorted to spending the rest of the visit talking with my new friend. I'd have to tell my editor we couldn't use the interview. The longer we'd spoken, the more farfetched his stories had become.

"I took out an army of men, over one hundred of 'em with my own bare hands!" he said, laughing.

His face lit up as he spoke. It was clear he would fade in and out of conversations. I watched him closely and you could almost see it. He would answer one question precisely and to the point and moments later struggle to find the easiest of words. A nurse walked in during our conversation and she lovingly moved the blanket that lay in his lap to cover his legs. He thanked her by name but minutes later had forgotten she'd come at all.

Before leaving, I thanked him for talking with me, and made my way to the hall. Standing at his doorway, I wished we'd met years earlier.

"Did you see my postcard?" he asked.

"No, I didn't; show it to me," I said as I walked over to the framed card beside his bed.

As I picked it up, he told me it was from a woman named Emma.

"She was the most beautiful lady you'd ever laid eyes on. She sent me that postcard on her wedding day," he chuckled. "She was all dressed up in a white wedding gown, about to say 'I do' and when the church doors opened for her to walk down the aisle to meet her groom, she slammed them shut! She ran back home, and sent me that card. She was my best friend growing up. She told me she'd be waiting 'til I got home from the army and we'd get married."

It was another of his stories. I was sure the postcard was significant in some way, but that was pretty farfetched.

As I pulled out of the nursing home, I called Mr. Walter's daughter from my car. I told her I'd visited her father and as much as I'd enjoyed talking with him, I couldn't publish the piece because of his condition.

She was kind and not surprised. She said her father's dementia had worsened over the last few months. But before we hung up, I told her what her dad said about defeating an army of German soldiers with his bare hands.

"That sounds just like him," she laughed.

I also went on to tell her about a postcard he'd shown me, and the story he'd shared of the woman, his childhood friend who'd stopped her wedding with minutes to spare and professed her love for him.

There was a pause on the other end of the phone. "Hello?"

"That one is true," she said, quietly.

She told me of the sixty-two-year marriage between her father and mother and how her mother waited for the soldier she'd always loved to return home from war.

"They had never even been on a first date," Mr. Walter's daughter said.

A week later I drove back to the nursing home and visited Mr. Walter again. He told me about Emma in great detail, never once trailing off as I'd witnessed days before. He recounted what Emma had worn the day he'd seen her upon his return, the address of their first home, their family pet, and Emma's favorite flowers he'd planted along the front porch stoop.

We published his story on the front page of the newspaper a week later. I hand delivered a copy to him.

"Why do you think you remembered so much about Emma, but so little about the war?" I asked.

He sighed, thinking for a moment, then told me, "World War II was a big part of my life, but Emma was the best part."

~Amanda Dodson

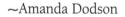

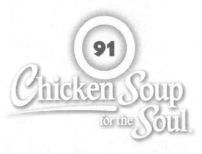

When Research Becomes a Passion

You can't live a perfect day without doing something for someone who will never be able to repay you.
~John Wooden

've been taking care of people with Alzheimer's disease for many years as a clinical research coordinator, managing trials for people with dementia. The relationships I build as I work with these individuals and their families are rewarding, but also challenging. Many of the studies I coordinate are long, from many months to several years, and over time I get to know the families quite well. But there always comes a time when I have to say goodbye.

I always wonder, do I tell them goodbye several times on different days and hope they remember? Or do I tell them once for the last time and that is that?

Some may ask: Why say goodbye when the study participants won't remember? Every time, my hope is that this may be the one time they do remember.

Then I realize that what I really care about is making sure they know I care about them. That is all that matters.

Bob and his wife were in one of my studies and had long, frequent visits to our study center. We had a common interest in skiing and soon found ourselves comparing Vermont mountains to Michigan mountains. We decided Vermont mountains were much better for skiing. They loved hearing about the progress of my niece, who was skiing for the first time for her high school team. We always had something to talk about during their visits.

As the study continued, I realized Bob was going downhill cognitively. It broke my heart. I had a hard time seeing such a previously vibrant man unable to speak in coherent sentences or recall my name. When the study came to a close, I prepared myself to say goodbye.

During Bob's last appointment, I hugged him. As I said goodbye, he stopped, turned, and smiled at me. I wondered if he understood what I was saying. His wife and I both made a promise to keep in touch. I tried not to let the tears fall but it just couldn't be helped.

As the year passed, Bob's wife kept me up to date on how he was doing, and it wasn't good. He continued to go downhill, slowly losing the ability to engage in some of his favorite activities. Through it all, Bob's wife amazed me with her constant cheerfulness, courage, and wisdom. I encouraged her to take care of herself so she could be there for Bob.

All too quickly, Bob's wife called to tell me he was now in a nursing facility. I know it was a difficult decision to make since she is so dedicated to her husband. Even with Bob no longer at home, she spends the greater part of each day with him and keeps in touch with me via e-mail. She said Bob smiles whenever she mentions my name. I know whenever I am in their area I have a place to visit, but it will also mean more goodbyes.

Will the goodbyes get easier as time passes? As I get older? Wiser? More experienced? Some people call Alzheimer's disease the longest goodbye and now I know why. Bob's story is not finished. There will be more goodbyes and none will be easy. Sometimes the tears are going to come and I can't stop them. We researchers become very attached to our "loved ones" as well, and our research becomes our passion, as we fight this disease along with those living with the disease and their families.

~Joanne L. Lord, LPN, BA, CCRC

Make sure your child knows that even though a person with dementia may be forgetful, love and kindness are still felt in the moment.

"Parent's Guide:
Helping Children and Teens Understand Alzheimer's Disease"
Alzheimer's Association

Living with Alzheimer's & Other Dementias

Chapter 11

The Special Bond with Grandchildren

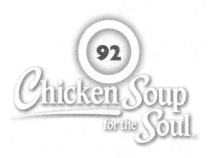

Understanding Nana

People who don't cherish their elderly have forgotten whence they came and whither they go.
~Ramsey Clark

t's funny, but even at a year and a half old, my second daughter is the spitting image of my grandmother. There are moments when Iris turns to me and I am gobsmacked by the likeness, made ready to banish any skepticism about reincarnation. Iris has Nana's smile, that rascally twinkle in her eye, and her mouth and brow take the same scrunched shape when she focuses on a tiny detail, like fitting a colored peg into the Lite-Brite.

Author Elizabeth Stone said about having children, "...it is momentous. It is to decide forever to have your heart go walking around outside your body." It is amazing to discover, or perhaps rediscover, that you can love and be loved so deeply. And every day I look at Iris, I am reminded of another unique love—between grandchild and grandparent.

As a kid, I was consumed with the anticipation of Nana's arrival for the holidays. I remember the feeling of her hug, breathing in her powdery perfume, sitting for hours at her feet while she brushed my hair. She'd marvel aloud at the many different shades of gold her painter's eye could see in my curly tresses. Nana couldn't get enough time with me, or I with her. Though I was one of four siblings, when I was alone with Nana, I felt like I was everything to her. She saved the locks of my freshly cut hair, the cards I made for her, my class photos, programs from school plays, all of which I later found when cleaning out her house. The hair was tucked in a beautiful silver box, labeled with my name and the various dates of my trims.

I've since held them up to my own daughter's head, and marveled at the colors. These days, I save neatly zip-locked locks from my daughter's haircuts, finger paintings, bathtime videos, in that desperate effort to freeze time. Like Nana, I'm attempting to grasp time as it slips through my fingers.

After dementia began to take hold of Nana, our relationship shifted. Occasional forgetfulness and confusion gave way to confounding outbursts of anger and paranoia. I remember a particularly brutal Christmas Eve, when there was no denying that I had become a stranger to her. I wore one of her fabulous Pucci print shirts with the express intention of amusing her. It was one of the many chic items she had happily handed down to me. When she saw me, her face tightened into a scowl, her eyes darted about and she accused me of stealing. I was an enemy. At the time I thought she was being unspeakably mean to me. I was unable to put myself in her shoes, and I was in denial about the road that lay ahead for Nana and all of us who were close to her.

Eventually, our holiday time together turned into rushed and guilt-ridden visits to the assisted living home. I'd re-comb Nana's hair, silently and unfairly cursing the nurses for styling it in a way Nana never would have approved. A ponytail? Seriously? Didn't they know she'd always choose elegant and sophisticated over cute or infantile? Didn't they read dissatisfaction on her face when she looked in the mirror?

I know she communicated with this overworked staff in fits and starts, in the dialog of a two-year-old, but did she have to suffer the indignity of being brushed off, rushed, misinterpreted, and spoken to like a toddler? She still had something to say, she still deserved to be heard.

Even though no one could understand her words, I always got the gist of what she was saying. I knew when Nana was joking with me. She'd get that devilish grin and tease me about how handsome my husband is, under her breath, with a requisite elbow jab, all in gibberish. Somehow I still knew when she was happy or sad, bothered or giddy. And yet I demonized the staff in my head, for not "getting" her, for not interacting with her as you would my charming, independent, sophisticated Nana. I did this even though it was this staff that did all the heavy lifting day in and day out, who dedicated their lives to caregiving, and to making sure all of Nana's needs were met every exhausting hour of the day.

On New Year's Day 2008 I brought my tiny firstborn daughter to see her. Nana was wearing a pink paper crown that said Happy New Year. This time I didn't silently curse the staff. It was actually kind of perfect—cheesy and perfect. A crown befitting the simple joy of childhood celebrations. A joy I was ready to reconnect with. The only "words" she uttered that day were various combos of "doo," "dee," and, "doe," and she had a tendency to sing them.

Nana was nervous and thrilled, overwhelmed, and amazed when she held baby Oona. Though she may not have been able to understand the concept that the baby had been born on her birthday, she seemed to grasp a deep kind of meaning. She "told" me that she was happy for me, that my little redheaded child was a wonder, was God's greatest gift, that she couldn't believe that her baby had this baby. She told me all that through her new language of sounds and tunes. Her language evaded everyone around her, but not me. Nana may have been losing the ability to speak, but I was relearning how to listen.

Any mother can attest to knowing what her child is saying, feeling, needing, even though the ability to speak has not yet been refined. I'm the master of translating for baby Iris, and I've seen friends wonder how the heck I knew she was asking for more butter, or requesting "Old MacDonald" over the "Itsy Bitsy Spider," when all she used was a random combo of, "buh," "la la" and "wee." Did my time with Nana help hone this skill? Every time I flex this Mom superpower, I'm reminded of that desire to protect Nana from being misunderstood. Boil it down, and I'm simply reminded of our basic human need to connect.

Nothing can prepare you for the grief of a loved one slipping away. There were incredibly hard days for Nana and my dad, and the rest of us. There was the suffering and fear and frustration at the onset, the stress of finding the right caregivers, the guilt of not having more time or resources.

As I experience Iris's little triumphs as she discovers speech, I'm reminded of Nana's gradual heartbreaking loss. Every day Iris reminds me of Nana. Shakespeare famously referred to the "seventh" and last "age" of life as "second childishness and mere oblivion," but it's not oblivion. In her own way, my grandmother knew and was known. Dementia and Alzheimer's inarguably rob us of so much, but they can't rob us of our most precious connections.

~Sarah Rafferty

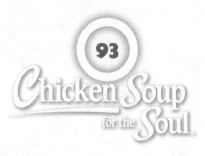

Out to Lunch

You will find as you look back upon your life that the moments
when you have truly lived are the moments
when you have done things in the spirit of love.
~Henry Drummond

The elevator doors slide open and I step into the fifth-floor lobby of the assisted living complex where my grandmother lives. DEMENTIA UNIT, the sign above the nursing station says. WELCOME!

There, in one of several wing-backed chairs scattered about the lobby, sits Grandmother. She is dressed in slacks and a flowered blouse and, although it's July and steamy hot outside, a heavy cardigan sweater. Her black patent leather purse rests on her lap.

"Hey, Grandmother," I say.

She looks at me and I spot a flash of recognition. "Jennie!" she says. "What are you doing here?"

"Today's Tuesday — the day we go out to lunch," I tell her, leaning down to kiss her cheek. "Remember? Just like every week." She nods. Near her, smiling pleasantly, is a woman I've never seen before.

"Hello," I say. The woman continues to smile but says nothing.

"This is my new best friend," Grandmother tells me, patting the woman's arm. "And this," she tells her friend, "is my nephew, Jennie."

I do not tell her that I'm not her nephew or her sister or her cousin or any of the other kinfolk she invariably imagines me to be. I am just grateful she recognizes me and remembers my name.

"Are you hungry?" I ask. Grandmother nods. I sign her out at the nurses' station but she hesitates before we step onto the elevator.

"I need to go back to my apartment. I forgot something."

"You have your purse and your sweater," I tell her. "What did you forget?"

"I need to be sure I turned off the stove."

We head down the hall to Grandmother's apartment. I don't tell her that all the stoves on the dementia floor are decoys, and not one of them is plugged in. I don't remind her that she doesn't cook in this apartment because three meals a day are provided in the dining room. I simply snap on the overhead light in the tiny kitchen and watch while she fiddles with the burner knobs, all of which are in the off position. She twists one of them to high. "There," she says. "That's better."

My car is parked about fifty yards from the front door of the complex and I ask Grandmother if she wants to wait while I get it. "No," she says. "I can walk." And she's right. She walks just fine for a woman who's almost eighty-eight years old, and I whisper a little prayer of gratitude for that.

I help her into the passenger seat. "Don't forget your seatbelt," I say. She stares at me with a blank look. I grab the chrome part of the buckle and hand it to her. "Pull this across your lap and snap it in." I walk around the car and slide behind the steering wheel. Grandmother is still holding the loose end of the seatbelt.

"I don't know what to do with this," she confesses. "So I'll just hold it."

I buckle her seatbelt and adjust the shoulder strap so that it's comfortable across her chest. "Now, what would you like for lunch?"

Grandmother is quiet for a long time and I wonder whether she's contemplating her choices or has simply forgotten the question. "Fried oysters," she finally says.

Fried oysters? In the fifty-something years I've known my grand-mother, I've never once seen her eat fried oysters or any other kind of seafood. I never knew she was aware there was such a thing as a fried oyster. But we're in a big city. I'll find a restaurant that serves them.

We're seated and the waitress hands us each a menu. Grandmother dutifully opens hers, though she can no longer make sense of the written word. "Look here," I say, pointing to the seafood column. "You can get a fried oyster platter or an oyster po' boy."

"Do they have meatloaf?"

Without meaning to, I sigh. "I thought you wanted fried oysters."

She frowns and shakes her head. "I don't like oysters."

So we order meatloaf and mashed potatoes and green beans. "And a cup of hot coffee," Grandmother tells the waitress. "I'm about to freeze to death. I think I must have low blood."

I smile to myself. Grandmother has been complaining of "low blood" for as long as I can remember, although—even when she didn't have dementia—she couldn't explain what that meant.

Our lunch is delicious and Grandmother eats every bite. Again, I whisper a prayer of thanks that her appetite is good.

As we head for home, Grandmother asks me to stop at the dollar store. She slowly pushes her cart up and down the aisles, staring in fascination at the hundreds of items on the shelves. "Is there something in particular you're looking for?" I ask.

"Toilet paper."

"Grandmother, they provide toilet paper at your apartment. Remember?"

"Well, I need some more," she insists. "I'm almost out."

We find the paper goods aisle and she picks out two packs of toilet paper and carefully puts them in the cart. On the way to the checkout lane, we pass a display of hair care products. Grandmother stops and slides a sparkly purple hairbrush off a hook. "This is pretty," she says.

"Do you need a new hairbrush?"

"Is that what this is?"

I nod.

"I don't know if I need one."

"Let's get it just in case," I say.

When we arrive back at the assisted living complex, we ride the elevator to the fifth floor. Grandmother's new best friend is still sitting in the same wing-backed chair, dozing softly. We don't wake her. I sign Grandmother in at the nurses' station and we make our way down the hall to her apartment. I open the door of the small linen closet and put the two new packages of toilet paper beside the half-dozen packages on the shelf. I remove the plastic wrapper from the sparkly purple hairbrush and set it next to the other hairbrushes on the bathroom counter.

It's time to tell Grandmother goodbye. She's in the kitchen, fiddling with the stove knobs.

"Good thing we got home when we did," she says. "My nurse left the stove on high. She could have burned the place down."

I give Grandmother a kiss. "I'll see you next Tuesday," I tell her. "We'll go out to lunch."

She puts her arms around me and hugs me tight. "Thanks for the oysters."

"You're welcome."

"I love you, Jennie," she says.

"I love you, too," I answer.

~Jennie Ivey

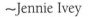

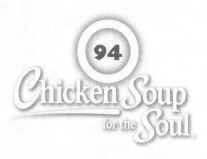

94

Joy in an Unexpected Friendship

It's one of nature's way that we often feel closer to distant generations than to the generation immediately preceding us.

~Igor Stravinsky

O ur entire family was over at my parents' house for Thanksgiving—the scene was the same each year. The eight grandchildren were running around playing, arguing and playing some more. The adults were finished with the meal, lazing in the living room on the good couches, which were always covered with an old quilt when my family came to visit. We sat there watching the Cowboys game, chatting and trying to keep my dad from steering the conversation to politics.

I had always found the similarities between my grandmother and my daughter, Lizzie, who has autism, fascinating. Lizzie was about four years old and did not interact much with anyone; neither did my grandmother. My grandmother's grip on reality had slowly been sucked out of her as Alzheimer's took its toll; similarly, Lizzie seemed to lack any understanding of our day-to-day lives.

Both Lizzie and my grandmother were often in their own worlds. Lizzie would flap her arms and loudly recite all the words from *Dora the Explorer*. My grandmother would rub some sort of fabric in between her fingers and read a script from an earlier time in her life when she still had young children at home. They both seemed to wander around the house with no sense of purpose.

As the adults were chatting, I realized things had gotten very quiet. Eerily quiet. Way too quiet. Lizzie had either gotten into something she wasn't supposed to, or gotten out of the house.

I immediately jumped up and began my search.

Kitchen? Nope.

Den? Not there.

Bathroom? Oops, wrong person. Sorry.

Then I heard it... the sweet sound of young and old giggling together. I peeked around the corner and what did I see? Lizzie and Grandma had found the remote control for the lamp in the bedroom. Such a simple thing; how could this possibly be bringing so much joy to both of them? They would walk into the bedroom, push the button, watch the light turn on and break out laughing.

After they completed their immediate cause-and-effect thrill, they would turn the light off, walk out, and then Lizzie would grab Grandma's hand and pull her back into the room again. They would repeat this simple act over and over, again and again and again. Each time the light flipped on, they would laugh hysterically as if they had never experienced this phenomenon before.

The repetition of the light made sense to Lizzie, and she had found her perfect playmate—my grandma, a sweet old lady with no short-term memory! This was truly an unexpected friendship that brought joy to both of them.

~Julie Hornok

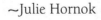

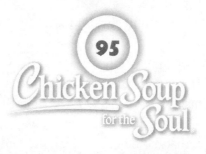

95

The Struggle for His Sanity

Grandchildren are the dots that connect the lines from
generation to generation.
~Lois Wyse

t was a cold January day and I walked into my grandfather's house for one of our normal visits. There was a scent of fresh leather from his new furniture. He greeted me with a warm smile.

"Hi honey," he said while he walked towards me with his arms slowly opening wide enough for me to fall into.

"Hey Papa, have you already had dinner?" I asked, slowly releasing our hug. "If not, I brought some leftovers."

As I walked over to the table to set down his food I noticed some peculiar things. Crackers were stored in the microwave and photos were evenly laid out on the table as if he had thought out exactly where each picture should go. Without responding, he shuffled his way over to the table next to me, gently picked up a picture of my mother when she was a child, and examined it.

With a quick glance I said, "Isn't that a cute picture of her?" Walking away to grab a plate he said something that broke my heart and terrified me.

"Yeah, it is. But why do I have this picture? Who is she?"

I turned around and saw an expression on his face that I will never forget. He looked genuinely lost. I saw no spark in his eyes, just a deep blue abyss.

That was the beginning of his fight, and the start of my struggle to keep him with me. At that moment I realized why my family was scared for him. This is what Alzheimer's was doing to him while I was at school, at practice, sleeping, and now, while I was standing right next to him. From that moment on, I took the initiative to help him. I stayed at his house most of the time for the next three years.

I did his laundry, cooked, cleaned, paid his bills, mowed the lawn, tucked him into bed at night, and laid his clothes out for the next day. If I didn't he would forget and wear the same outfit for days. I brushed his teeth, helped him into the shower, rubbed his feet, and rolled him around town in his wheelchair so he could socialize. I'd buy his groceries, and give him his medicine. Every day for me was dancing in circles, doing the same thing, but it was a spontaneous adventure for him.

During my time caring for him, I grew from a thirteen-year-old girl whose only focus was to make myself happy, to a sixteen-year-old young woman who had to grow up and take responsibility for someone else's life.

I learned to be compassionate, patient, and understanding to make someone else content. I had to be his light when he couldn't see where he was going. I had to hold his hand when he was scared. When he was crying because he didn't understand what was happening to him I embraced him, even though I couldn't explain what was happening to him either.

Then it happened. I came home from work, ready to do my second job. "Hey Papa," I said, walking up to the table to set down his to-go dinner and my purse. I turned around just as his fist was about to hit me.

"Who are you? Get out of my house!" he screamed at me, taking another step toward me, shaking with fear. His eyes were mean.

"Grandpa, stop! It's Amy. I take care of you!" There was an uneasy silence. He just stood there examining me. Not taking the chance, I backed another step away.

"Grandpa, do you remember me? I live with you. I'm Amy!" I was trying to find a flicker of remembrance in his eyes, but saw nothing. He was so deadly serious it sent chills up my spine.

Standing there breathing hard, he pointed to the door and in a shaky voice said, "Get Out!"

That was the first time I'd ever looked at my grandpa and saw the monster that was slowly killing him. The monster that destroyed his laugh, his will to sing, his enthusiasm for life and the love he used to have for me. With tears in my eyes, and a knot in my throat, I turned away and left. Feeling defeated, the next day my family took him to a nursing home.

He died a few months later. I grew up a lot during those years and I don't regret the time I spent caring for him. I couldn't control the fact that my grandpa was losing himself, and eventually didn't even know me, his caregiver, but I could control how I treated him. I let him know he would always have me by his side no matter what. I am so happy that I could do this for him.

~Amy Merrill

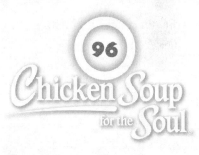

96

Still My Grammy

Grandma always made you feel she had been waiting to see just you all day and now the day was complete.

~Marcy DeMaree

My grandmother was diagnosed with the early stages of Alzheimer's disease when I was in fifth grade. At that point in my life, I was a kid. I was selfish as all kids are, so I didn't think twice about it. I had no idea how it would eventually affect my life, as well as my family, in such a large way.

I have a very tight-knit family, and my grammy is the glue that holds us together. I remember going to my grandparents' farmhouse every moment I could when I was a kid. My grammy would always make me chocolate milk and a peanut butter and Fluff sandwich. We would watch *Winnie the Pooh* movies and color—my grammy and I both love the smell of a new box of crayons. Sometimes, if I were lucky, she would take me to the barn to feed the calves or to see the new kittens. Little did I know, these would be the memories of my childhood that I would miss the most.

As I grew up, I noticed my grammy changing. At first, it was just little things. She would forget where she set her book, or she couldn't find her purse. Once again, I didn't think it was serious. I could never have guessed how it would progress, transforming my grammy into someone I could hardly recognize.

There was one incident in particular that was my wake-up call.

I remember thinking, "This isn't a joke, and my grammy isn't my grammy anymore. This is a serious disease."

About three years ago, a tornado went through our town. Although it was heading straight for my grandparents' farmhouse, it died down before destroying my childhood sanctuary. My father and I went to visit my grandparents the day after the storm, just to make sure they were okay. I went inside to find Grammy. I gave her a hug and took my regular seat on the couch across from her. We passed the time by talking for hours on end, about anything and everything that was on our minds. The power was out, and it got dark in what seemed like a matter of minutes.

Then, Grammy turned to me, and with empty eyes that stared right past me, asked, "Now you're graduating this year, aren't you?" I was a freshman, so I was confused why she was asking me about graduation. Grammy was the type of person who could tell you the exact date and time when every one of her grandchildren came into this world. Her innocent question caught me off guard. I assured her that no, I was not yet a senior; I still had a few years until graduation, and casually moved the conversation along.

Soon, my father asked if I was ready to go home. I silently nodded my head yes, and we headed out. As soon as I got into the car, I started to cry. My father asked me what was wrong, and all I could manage to blurt out was, "Is Grammy going to be at my graduation?"

It took him a long time to come up with a response, and when he finally did, I heard the sadness in his voice. "Yes. She may not know where she is, but she will be there, no matter what." I looked at my father, and I saw a tear running down his cheek. I had never seen him cry. The rest of the car ride home was silent. When we finally arrived home, I went straight to my room. I locked my door and I cried for hours. That night made me realize that things were going to start changing fast.

Ever since that talk with my grammy, I have matured and stepped up. Her Alzheimer's has progressed to about stage 3 now. She is at the point that she can't see what is directly in front of her. When I see her get that look that says, "I don't know where I am or what I am doing," it's my automatic response to help her by getting her a plate of food or easing her into a chair.

At first, I didn't notice the strange looks I got from the other members of my family. Then, last summer, when I was cutting Grammy's food at a family picnic, I looked up and saw all my aunts, uncles and cousins looking at me. I just ignored them for the moment and went back to helping Grammy. Later on, I asked my mother why they looked at me like that. She explained that they still picture my grandmother as the one who takes care of everyone else. They had not yet realized that the roles had switched; after years of being the sole caregiver of the family, she was the one who needed their help.

Now, at sixteen, I have a better understanding of Alzheimer's disease. My grammy's deterioration has had a huge impact on my family and has put a lot of stress on us all. It greatly upsets me to know that one day Grammy will no longer be able to look at me and say, "That is my granddaughter, Kayla."

At my graduation, when I am sitting on the stage waiting to receive my diploma, I will look out over the crowded gym and see Grammy there, sitting with the rest of my family. She may not understand what is going on, but she will be there. After the ceremony, I will find Grammy in the huge swarm of people, and I will hug her. I know she will forget me someday, but I am not dwelling on that fact. For now, I try to cherish the good days and to get through the bad days as best I can. She will always be my grammy and I will always be her granddaughter.

~K. Thorp

Author's note: Since the original version of this story was written in 2011, I graduated from high school. I am happy to report that I was able to give my grammy a hug as I walked out of the gym. As my father promised, she made it to my graduation.

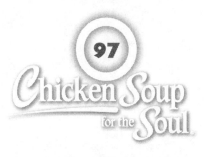

97

Pretty Little Heaven

He who sings frightens away his woes.
~*Miguel de Cervantes*, Don Quixote

When two people truly love each other, it is hard for one to imagine life without the other. I believe this was the case for my grandmother, Abuela Hilda. My grandparents met when they were teenagers in Havana, Cuba, got married young and had been inseparable ever since. They had three strapping young boys, the eldest being my father. After the Cuban Revolution, they left everything behind and moved to Miami, Florida to pursue a better life. They lived a humble life and always made sure the house was filled with love.

Many years later, my grandfather died of lung cancer and shortly after my grandmother started showing symptoms of Alzheimer's disease. My sisters and I were fairly young, so for a while we were unaware of what was happening to Abuela. We loved her and would always visit her on Sundays, spending the day talking, laughing and—my personal favorite—singing together. Although we're Cuban, she would often sing "Cielito Lindo," a popular Ranchera song from Mexico. The chorus goes like this: "Ay, ay, ay, ay. Canta y no llores/ Porque cantando se alegran/ Cielito lindo, los corazones." ["Ay, ay, ay, ay. Sing and don't cry. Because singing gladdens, pretty little heaven, the hearts."]

Abuela had a slow decline. What at first seemed like simple forgetfulness became alarming when she looked at my dad and asked,

"Who are you?" I had fewer and fewer conversations with her and her temper got progressively worse. My dad was a trouper throughout. He remained so strong and stoic that sometimes we didn't realize how serious it was. We watched her shift between recognition and confusion until the day came when she stopped being aware that she even had memory problems.

The notion that my abuela had Alzheimer's disease didn't hit home until one Sunday while we were all talking in the back yard. I was making a joke and trying to get her to laugh when she began screaming at my sisters and me, calling us names and demanding to know why we were in her house. No amount of begging and pleading could make her recognize us again. She had passed the point of no return.

Sometimes she would think she was back in Cuba, going to see a friend and we would find her wandering in the middle of the street. We hired a live-in caregiver to make sure she was safe, and to feed, dress, and bathe her.

Conversations with Abuela grew shorter and shorter until eventually she just sat in her rocking chair as we all took turns trying to engage her. Every now and then she would say a few words and everyone would stop to listen. But best was when out of the blue she would begin singing "Cielito Lindo." "Ay Ay Ay Ay/Canta y no llores…" Did she know what she was singing? Was she trying to tell us something? Was this perhaps all the comfort she could muster to offer my father and the rest of us? She had forgotten her name, her family, and even how to perform basic bodily functions, yet was able to sing this timeless song with ease.

Our last few weeks together were unspeakably sad. Even the indomitable armor that my dad seemed to don finally cracked and I saw him cry for the first time in my life. On her hospital bed, her tender body lay motionless and her curly hair lightly framed her surprisingly piercing green eyes. We stayed by her side, holding her hand until the very end. Days would go by where she wouldn't say a word. At this point, she seemed to have forgotten everything. Her body and mind had failed her, and yet oddly enough, the only thing she seemed to remember was that familiar song as her frail voice floated through the hospital halls. "Ay Ay Ay Ay, Canta y no llores..." Was there a tiny piece of her fighting until the very end, a small voice struggling to be heard amidst the fog of dementia? Was this perhaps the song she and my grandfather would dance to?

I'll never know. She was seventy-six when she passed away on Valentine's Day.

The memory of Abuela's voice singing that song still echoes deep within my soul. I grew up to be a singer among other things, and if that song was her last message to us then her legacy lives on. When given the choice to sing or to cry, I think of my Abuela, and I sing.

~Yvette Gonzalez-Nacer

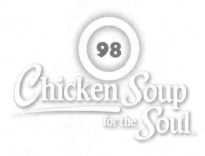

98

All You Need Is Love

To us, family means putting your arms around each other and being there.
~Barbara Bush

When I heard that my grandmother, already in poor health, had been diagnosed with Alzheimer's, I had no idea what to expect. Beyond what I'd read in books and heard through word-of-mouth I knew very little about the disease.

I live abroad and had been planning a trip back that would include a visit with my grandmother. In preparation of what I feared I would find, I read up on Alzheimer's and talked to friends who had relatives with the disease. Having nursed my mother through to the end of a terminal illness, a part of me feared a repeat of that pain. I almost didn't want to go.

My uncle and his son live with my grandmother—my cousin was attending classes in the early morning or evening and taking care of our grandmother the rest of the time. My cousin is several years younger than me, in his early twenties—he loves his Pit Bull, fixing his vintage car, and listening to music. He's a great guy, but he sports a large tattoo and loves his beer, so he wasn't exactly what I'd call a classic nurturer.

While I was there, I told my cousin and uncle to take as much time off as they wanted while I stayed with my grandmother.

We had a wonderful visit. I cooked her special meals, cleaned some neglected corners of the house, and accompanied her and my uncle on a doctor's visit. Some days she remembered me; some days she didn't. One day I startled her badly when she awoke in the late morning to go to the bathroom and, only half awake, saw me in her living room. She thought I was a visitor and felt terrible that I'd been left on my own and no one was entertaining me. I reassured her and we carried on. I told myself that this wasn't so bad after all.

Then one night it was. Grandma had stayed up a little too late, perhaps, and she got emotional when she couldn't figure out where her bedroom was. It wasn't the first time that she had trouble finding her bedroom or bathroom but this time she lay down on her bed and cried: "What's wrong with me? Am I losing my mind? Why can't I remember that? Should I go to a home?"

I stood in the doorway feeling completely clueless, old fears from seeing my mother in pain flooding over me. I tried to think of what to do, what to say, but drew a blank.

From behind me I heard my cousin walk quietly past me into the dimly-lit room. Gently he lay down next to Grandma. "It's okay. Don't cry, Old One [his name for her]. This is your house, and you're going to stay right here for as long as you want to. It'll be okay."

Deeply touched, I backed out of the room as her crying subsided.

Fifteen minutes my later, my cousin emerged. "She just needs a little reassurance sometimes when she gets confused," he said simply, and smiled.

Just a little love. I stood in awe of this unlikely caregiver. Truly, Grandma had the best care ever — someone who loved her.

~Evangeline Neve

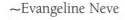

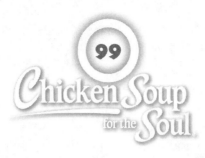

Fade to Black

Love is like dew that falls on both nettles and lilies.
~Swedish Proverb

She can't remember the last time she saw him, though it was only three years ago. It was on July 3rd, a hot, moonless summer night, and she'd spent the final moments holding his hand, alternately speaking to him in hushed tones and singing "Let Me Call You Sweetheart" ever so softly into his ear, her cheek meeting his where it lay on the stiff hospital pillow.

But she can tell you how they met, in vivid Technicolor detail: about the pouring rain that day some seventy years ago when her big brother brought him to the house, a drowned rat by all appearances. But even so, she couldn't take her eyes off his; the way they twinkled and danced! Just one look, and before she knew it she was following him into happily ever after.

She can't remember the name of the nice lady who fed her lunch yesterday and breakfast this morning; the one who cajoles her into taking "just one more bite"; the one who brings the Styrofoam cup of too-sweet lemonade to her lips to wash it down; the one who is a mere child herself, but inevitably crows about what a "good girl" she's been to eat so much of the pureed food that passes as a meal these days.

She will ask you, though, about your babies, and even about Ms. Stinky-Son, her great-grandson's not-so-favorite kindergarten teacher. She'll ask if "that woman" ever gave him back his truck, recalling an incident long forgotten by the parties involved. Her voice is animated as she stands ready to defend the shaggy-haired five-year-old with the tear-stained face of a decade or more ago, standing before her mind's eye in a twisted version of the here and now.

She can't remember why she doesn't see you every day, or, perhaps more aptly put, that she doesn't. Where has everybody gone? Why is she in this awful godforsaken place? She hates it here, she says, without saying a word, but still, you can read the indictment on her face. She wants to go home. Can't you take her there? Sit on the big flagstone back porch and gaze across the river, have a glass of tea and talk about remember when? The pleading that goes unsaid is enough to break a heart in two, jagged edges still piercing and pinching long after the visit is over.

She won't remember that you've been here, almost as quickly as you go. Tomorrow, today will be just yesterday, those short-term memories the first attacked by the cruel, unforgiving scourge that wipes the surface of her mind clean each night.

But I'll remember.

"I have to go, Grandma. I'll be back soon."

Her face turns, seeking mine.

"I love you," I say, nearly choking on the emotion welling up.

Her cloudy eyes find mine, and lock there in a long, present moment.

"I love you, sweetie," she states with all the authority of the grandmother I've always known. "And don't you ever forget it."

~Jennifer Waggener

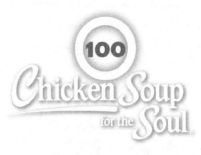

A Beautiful Tragedy

Life is a shipwreck but we must not forget to sing in the lifeboats.
~Voltaire

"Out of the mouths of babes," a biblical phrase, refers to the sometimes surprising brilliance of a child's perspective. So it was when my twelve-year-old granddaughter accompanied me on a visit to see my mom. Mom had been diagnosed with Alzheimer's several years earlier. I made the 250-mile drive to visit her every month or so, and the changes in her memory and behavior were subtle to me. But my granddaughter hadn't seen her in months, and the changes shocked her.

Mother never made the connection to our identities. She didn't know I was her son, didn't know I had brought her great-granddaughter to see her. One of her regular patterns was to point at a photo on the wall and say, "See my family? I had a great big, wonderful family."

The photo was one taken at her home thirty years earlier, and there she was, seated in a chair, with all four of her children behind her. The decorations showed clearly that we had gathered for a Christmas at her home.

My granddaughter was unusually quiet on the long drive home. Normally a loquacious girl, she stared out the window at the Texas landscape for much of the four-hour drive. When she spoke, it was to ask questions about Mom, like, "What was her marriage like?" Or, "Was she a happy person?"

It was strange, fielding these questions from a twelve-year-old, and stranger still that she seemed so affected by our visit. She wiped a tear now and then, as did I. I was surprised at hers. My tears were because I knew my mother had lost eighty years worth of wonderful memories. I didn't think my granddaughter had the life experience to appreciate that.

A few weeks later I was invited to go hear my granddaughter perform at a music café. She was a budding songwriter, and a decent musician at age twelve, and I loved watching her few opportunities to shine in public. When it was her turn, she announced that she had written a song in honor of my mother—a surprise. The song was called "That Same December."

The song was sweet, and one of its phrases, "you feel there's something to remember, always stuck in that same December," was so poignant I was choking back tears. The lyrics took me back to the phrase: "out of the mouths of babes."

I had worried about my granddaughter's comprehension of Mother's disease, worried about her moodiness on the way home, wondered if the visit presented questions about life too tough for a twelve-year-old mind.

But her lyrics put things in better perspective than I had been able to:

"A well-kept heart, but a broken mind,
Thoughts so lost, too hard to find,
Memories dissolve away each broken heart and your wedding day,
You can't recall any suffering,
Oh, what a beautiful tragedy."

In that moment, in that song, I found such hope and inspiration. I had cried because Mom couldn't remember her family that loved her, couldn't recall her wedding day, but I realized that she also couldn't recall any suffering.

She was a good, loving woman, faithful to my father, loyal to her family. I needed to be taken back to her well-kept heart, and stop seeing only her broken mind.

A twelve-year-old helped me see that Alzheimer's can, in fact, be a beautiful tragedy.

~Danny Carpenter

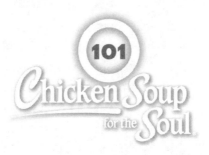

No Longer a Thief

*Nobody can do for little children what grandparents do. Grandparents sort of
sprinkle stardust over the lives of little children.*

~Alex Haley

My grandma was now a tiny version of herself, but even on days when she was trapped deep within the fog of dementia, the best parts of Grandma were still there. She may not have known our names, and she mistook her son for her precious husband whom she mourned terribly, but she was a sweet, happy lady always bringing smiles to the staff and fellow residents where she lived.

We were all experiencing a great loss—she was right in front of us, yet, she wasn't. She was lost in the recesses of her mind, her memories jumbled, faces and names confused. I wanted desperately for my preschool daughter to know my grandma. The tricky part was that my daughter experiences autism. How would I bridge the gap between loved one and stranger, seventy-something and five-year-old, a person who experiences dementia and a person who experiences autism?

I knew that when we introduced the two, my daughter would need to stay busy. I never take her anywhere without a well-packed activity bag. I also thought that my grandma might enjoy participating in the fun, so I packed for two.

The bag had treasured favorites like beads, pipe cleaners, crayons, paints, Play-Doh and other activities. From the moment my beloved grandma set eyes on my daughter she was enchanted by her every move. I stood back and watched my grandma beam. She wasn't quite sure who this little girl was, but she loved her all the same.

We found a table and set up our activities. Grandma eagerly participated, and though she was slower and her response times delayed, she gave every activity a try. But most of all she loved just being with her great-granddaughter and absorbing her youth and innocence.

I watched the two people I loved dearly and took mental snapshots of these precious moments. I watched as Grandma's worn hands brushed my daughter's hands, who was just beginning her life, and I watched as Grandma held on as long as my daughter would allow.

The irony of their social dance did not escape my notice. It didn't matter that my daughter couldn't make eye contact with Grandma, and it wasn't important to my daughter that my Grandma couldn't remember her name. For this moment in time, they were secret friends in a pretend tree house giggling and creating and just enjoying each other's presence. It didn't matter that they were scores of years apart in age, or that their social skills were terribly lacking; they had found common ground in shared activities and being friends. The absence of details and specifics that had built walls between so many others and had caused them to fall away, were the very glue that made this new, beautiful friendship work.

The absence of judgment and expectation was freeing for these two friends. They could make up stories, or speak in echolalia and neither one of them was offended, impatient, or annoyed. It became part of the dialogue.

The staff marveled, and everyone who watched this exchange, from nurses to other family to visitors, were charmed and touched to witness this precious new friendship bloom. While the friendship was nurtured and grew deeper it became increasingly more difficult with each visit to continue with the same activities. The hugs lasted longer, photos were taken, and the two friends were oblivious to what the rest of us knew was coming.

When Grandma passed away on a cold January day, I lost a beloved mentor and icon, a once strong and confident woman who taught me so much by her example and faith, and someone who loved me in the worst of times. But I also experienced my five-year-old daughter's loss of one of the most precious friendships she will ever experience—a friendship based on charm and whimsy, no expectations or judgment, and freedom to be exactly who God made her (and my grandma) to be.

Often, autism and dementia are viewed as thieves—faceless villains who steal and destroy. But in this story, autism and dementia were not the enemy; they were stepping stones to a beautiful and rare friendship.

~Amy L. Stout

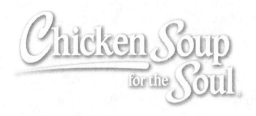

Afterword

Toni Morrison said, "If there's a book you really want to read, but it hasn't been written yet, then you must write it." We are so fortunate that here at Chicken Soup for the Soul we can do just that—see a need and fill it!

This book, for people who have been diagnosed with Alzheimer's or other dementias, and for their caregivers and loved ones, provides the kind of support and advice that we believe is delivered best through storytelling. After all, mankind has been passing on wisdom through storytelling for thousands of years. I think we all learn best when we hear real stories from real people who have already "been there, done that," so that's what we have provided you in this collection—personal stories, best practices, coping strategies and tips from one hundred people, each facing Alzheimer's or dementia from a different point of view. I'm sure you learned a lot and found stories that were particularly applicable to your situation.

And we are happy that we are able to support the good work of the Alzheimer's Association with this book. More than half the story contributors asked us to give their writing fees to the Alzheimer's Association, and all royalties from the book will go to the Association to continue its work. You can read about the Alzheimer's Association's programs throughout this book, as many of the story writers talk about what the Association has done for them and their families.

We are lucky that we have a variety of vehicles with which to raise money for worthy causes—our books, our comfort food line, our pet food, and our other products. Charitable giving has been a big part of Chicken Soup for the Soul's mission throughout its twenty-year history.

Last year, we published *Chicken Soup for the Soul: Raising Kids on the Spectrum*, with a portion of the proceeds going to the Kennedy Krieger Institute, which helps children and adolescents with disorders of the brain, spinal cord and musculoskeletal system, including autism. That book provides much needed support and advice to parents of children diagnosed with autism and Asperger's. And later this year, we will publish *Chicken Soup for the Soul: Recovering from Traumatic Brain Injuries*. Millions of people in the United States have suffered TBIs, whether from military service, sports, or accidents. That book will have a foreword by Lee Woodruff and proceeds from book sales will help the Bob Woodruff Foundation in its work with veterans.

We don't just give money to organizations that support research and care of people with brain injuries or disorders. Last year we also published *Chicken Soup for the Soul: Think Positive for Kids*, with royalties going to my coauthor Kevin Sorbo's children's education program, and we are also using proceeds from the 20th Anniversary Edition of *Chicken Soup for the Soul* to benefit several charities, including the Humpty Dumpty Institute. Humpty Dumpty runs programs all over the world promoting literacy, fighting poverty, disease and hunger, and enabling conservation programs for animals. Chicken Soup for the Soul provides support to Humpty Dumpty through all its books and other products.

This book about Alzheimer's is the biggest collaboration we have done so far with a non-profit. The idea came about when I was a speaker last year at a book festival that benefited the Alzheimer's Association. Kristen Cusato, then the Southwest Regional Director of the Alzheimer's Association Connecticut Chapter, was there and she spoke beautifully about her mother, who had dementia with Lewy bodies. Kristen connected me to the Association's national office and we started to develop the plan for this book. Kristen's own wisdom is passed along to you in this book in story 18, which starts off Chapter 3.

Then I met Cristin Marandino, the editor of *Greenwich Magazine*, who lost her mom to Alzheimer's three years ago, at age 74. Cristin is very active in the Alzheimer's Association and she furthered my resolve to help this wonderful organization and all the people affected by Alzheimer's by collaborating on this book. I'd like to share an excerpt from a speech that Cristin gave at a benefit she chaired for the Alzheimer's Association Connecticut Chapter last year:

> *My mother was the most giving person I will ever meet, so to see so much taken from her was heartbreaking.*
>
> *Alzheimer's is an insidious disease. It crept in and slowly robbed my mom of her memory and eventually her personality. But the most painful thing is that she knew. She knew she was slipping away and that there was absolutely nothing she could do to prevent it.*
>
> *Imagine being trapped under water, just beneath the surface. Your lungs are constricted and you can't breathe, but you know — and can see — that just a few inches away there is oxygen. If you could only get to the surface. Imagine the helplessness and fear you would feel. That level of suffering is unacceptable.*
>
> *The Alzheimer's Association is helping break through the surface. They are educating healthcare workers, providing care and services and funding the research. They are a lifeboat in a very scary storm.*
>
> *One gift I was given was the ability to be with my mom at the end of her battle. She had been in intensive care for ten days and was in and out of consciousness. She had not spoken for days. It became clear that it was time to bring in hospice so that she could leave the suffering behind.*
>
> *When the hospice nurses arrived, she was very aware that they were there and that it meant we gave our permission for her to move on. The doctors said that it would be at least a few days until she passed away. Just two hours after the hospice nurses arrived, my mother opened her eyes and looked at us and said: "I love you."*

She then literally took her last breath.

I share this because it is a powerful reminder. It is a reminder that although Alzheimer's robs its victims of so much, it does not — and can not — rob them of their spirit.

Cristin's speech is a powerful reminder of why we are all working so hard to make life better for those affected by Alzheimer's and other dementias, and why we are putting so many resources into finding a cure. With this book, we at Chicken Soup for the Soul are making our own small contribution to this cause.

~Amy Newmark
Publisher and Author
Chicken Soup for the Soul

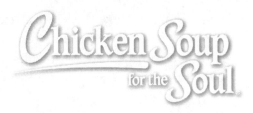

Meet Our Contributors

Kristina Aste-Mayer is an English teacher, yearbook advisor, and accompanist at Danvers High School. She majored in Music/English, minored in Philosophy, and united them in her Dante essay, "Music as Mirror," published in *Elements*, a research journal. She has a B.A. and M.Ed. degree from Boston College. Thanks to JP, family, friends!

Kris Bakowski lives in Athens, GA with her husband. They have one son. Kris enjoys speaking to groups around the country on a regular basis about her experiences with Alzheimer's. She also works in advocacy on a state and national basis, and serves on the Board of Governors for the Alzheimer's Association Georgia Chapter.

Rosemary Barkes won the Erma Bombeck Writing Competition at age sixty-four and has been writing ever since. She holds a Bachelor of Arts, Bachelor of Science, plus a Master of Science degree. Her recent book, *The Dementia Dance: Maneuvering Through Dementia While Maintaining Your Sanity*, has received rave reviews.

Nancy King Barnes is a registered practicing nurse who lives with husband in Rowlett, TX. Chicken Soup for the Soul has served as a wonderful venue to express her life's experiences that God has provided. Writing is a hobby and she is thankful to this publication for allowing her to share her heart.

Mike Belleville is a father of three, grandfather of three living and one that has passed on (love you Ethan). He is married to the most beautiful lady in the world and served twelve years in the Rhode Island Air National Guard with his dad and two brothers. Mike is grateful for having the best friends a guy can have and for knowing Michelle.

A graduate of Kent State University, **Lois Bennett** spent many years as a special education administrator and later worked with senior citizens, many with Alzheimer's, in nursing homes. Now living in Central Florida, she enjoys writing and editing books. She wrote *Essays: On Living with Alzheimer's Disease, The First Twelve Months*.

Nancy Stearns Bercaw lives in Vermont with her husband and son. Her work has appeared in publications from *The New York Times* to the *Korea Herald*. Her book, *Brain in a Jar: A Daughter's Journey through Her Father's Memory*, was published by Broadstone Books in April 2013. She is working on a second memoir about life as a mermaid.

Louise Harris Berlin holds master's degrees in history and broadcasting and is a long-time copywriter and editor. She and her husband, recent empty nesters, are enjoying the good life in Boise, ID. Her interests include quilting, writing, golf, travel and playing bocce in a summer league.

Maria Montagna Bohlman raised two children with her husband Rick. They have three grandchildren. She and her husband created The King's Pines, rental cabins they built in the Adirondack foothills. Maria enjoys writing, collecting beach glass, and rock painting. E-mail her at Agapeblue98@msn.com.

W. Bond received her Bachelor of Arts and master's degree from Lewis & Clark College. Wendy is a retired teacher and enjoys volunteering, sewing, cooking, and spending time with family and friends.

Dr. Bordisso was diagnosed with younger-onset Alzheimer's disease in 2010. He is a licensed marriage and family therapist, author, and inspirational speaker. As such, Bordisso speaks nationwide at conferences and conventions about mindful and spiritual living with Alzheimer's disease.

Jill Burns lives in the mountains of West Virginia with her wonderful family. She's a retired piano teacher and performer. She enjoys writing, music, gardening, nature, and spending time with her grandchildren.

Jean Salisbury Campbell, a retired school psychologist, wife and mother, graduated from the University of Florida and FIU, where she also studied creative writing. Caring for her mother during her six-year Alzheimer's decline propelled Jean to write about the priceless lessons learned that helped her cope with the loss.

Danny Carpenter is a Texas pastor, author/writer, Vietnam veteran, proud father of two daughters, and prouder grandfather of three. He enjoys golfing and family ski trips, strumming the ukelele, and writing with a passion.

Angie Carrillo has been a caregiver to her husband John since his diagnosis with Alzheimer's in 2008 at the age of sixty. Until then they lived a full life, filled with family, travel, and laughter. Angie writes to give others a peek at how she strives to balance full-time employment with caring for John and finding time for herself.

Kala Cota lives in a small logging community in Oregon. She teaches preschool and enjoys spending time with her husband, two grown children and new granddaughter. Since her mother's diagnosis, she is incredibly grateful for the support and encouragement from family and friends. Every journey is better when shared.

Linda Veath Cox lives in southern Illinois with the Bone Mafia—her two mixed breed mutts. A retired secretary from the Illinois

Department of Natural Resources, she has had short stories and devotions published and is a regular contributor to "Divine Detour" (http://kathyharrisbooks.com/blog).

Tracy Crump has published thirteen Chicken Soup for the Soul stories. She also edits *The Write Life* e-newsletter, writes a column for *Southern Writers Magazine*, and enjoys teaching other writers at conferences and through her Write Life Workshops. But her most important job is Grandma to three-year-old Nellie.

Carmen Cruz was born in a pueblo in Puerto Rico and was the youngest of eight siblings. At a young age, she discovered a passion for literature. Carmen's family is her pride and joy; she has two children and six grandchildren. At seventy-seven years old, Carmen dedicates her time to activities that exercise her mind.

After twenty-two years in TV news, **Kristen Cusato** made a life and career change when her mother Linda was diagnosed with Lewy Body Dementia. She worked for the Alzheimer's Association Connecticut Chapter as she cared for her mother. Kristen went back into TV after Linda passed, and works to end Alzheimer's.

Dr. David Davis has been practicing chiropractic in Connecticut since 1982. David loves teaching people in his community about health, and he also loves music, the outdoors and traveling the back roads of America on his Harley Davidson.

Martha Deeringer writes for children and adults from the back porch of her home on a central Texas cattle ranch. Visit her website at www.marthadeeringer.com.

Amanda Dodson is a wife and mother to three children: Grace, Garrett and Luke. She is a freelance writer and newspaper reporter for *The Stokes News* in North Carolina. Read her blog at amandatdodson.com.

Ginny Dubose has worked in senior housing for fifteen years, caring for seniors and helping their families with the day-to-day issues of the elderly. A graduate of Florida Southern College, Ginny is living her dream life with husband Ray and her sons, Dan and Alex, in sunny central Florida.

Cheryl Edwards-Cannon has been a giver of care for more than ten years and is currently writing a book about her experience. She is also a Care Consultant to those who are struggling with the challenges of elderly care. E-mail Cheryl at clearpathpartners14@gmail.com.

Linda Rose Etter taught for thirty-six years. She finished her Master of Arts in Biblical Studies in 2005. Her devotional book, *Listen To HIS Heartbeat*, was published in 2011. It contains seventy-five devotions that are humorous analogies and include scripture. She also has stories in three anthologies. Learn more at www.etterlinda.com.

Jean Ferratier, a Chicken Soup for the Soul regular, loves writing personal memoirs. A retired teacher, she is an active Present-Moment, Heart-Centered Life Coach. Her recent book is *Reading Symbolic Signs: How to Connect the Dots of Your Spiritual Life*. She loves dancing. She blogs at www.synchronousmoments.wordpress.com.

Kristi Cocchiarella FitzGerald has degrees in English and Theater and pursued graduate work in costumes until she realized she'd rather be writing. She lives in a place of spectacular beauty where she shares her life with her rugged Montana fisherman, their two Shih Tzus, Panda and Koala, and a diva cat named Moose.

Jennifer L. Freed treasures the stained and handwritten index cards her grandmother wrote recipes on. She has written a poetry chapbook, *These Hands Still Holding* (Finishing Line Press, 2014), and her poems have appeared in *The Cancer Poetry Project 2*, *The Healing Muse*, *JAMA*, and other publications. Learn more at Jfreed.weebly.com.

Susan Hanna Frook has firsthand knowledge of the challenges of Alzheimer's. She and her husband were raising their second family of three adopted children when the signs of this disease began to manifest in her husband. Frook hopes her story will bring encouragement to others who face living with Alzheimer's.

Elizabeth Parker Garcia teaches Communication Studies at the University of Texas-Pan American. When she is not teaching, she loves writing for children. Her father was fifty-two years old when she was born, so she is a member of the "sandwich generation" helping an aging parent while also serving her family as a mother and wife.

Molly Godby lives with her family of four in Zionsville, IN. She received a B.A. in Psychology, with a concentration in Elementary Education, from Randolph-Macon Woman's College in 1997. In 2007, her mother was diagnosed with dementia with probable onset of Alzheimer's. Read her blog at www.abundantlyawesome.blogspot.com.

Yvette Gonzalez-Nacer is a Cuban-American songwriter, singer, multi-instrumentalist, actress and humanitarian. She is best known for her work on the Emmy Award-winning series *The Fresh Beat Band* (Kiki) and just published her first children's book, *The Adventures of Little Eva*, which celebrates the importance of being yourself.

Rose M. Grant has a Master of Science in biology and is certified in Health Care Ethics. She recently retired from teaching. Her story is based on her manuscript, *I Left My Memory on a Bus Somewhere*, a compilation of dairies kept by Rose and her husband. Rose spends much of her time working with caregivers and the Alzheimer's Association.

Patty Gunnett had a lifelong dream of being a published author. After raising two sons and babysitting in churches, she achieved her goal by having five childhood stories published in the *Pittsburgh Post-*

Gazette. She now spends time writing and visiting her husband in the memory care center. E-mail her at patbob241@comcast.net.

Cynthia Guzman was a nurse for thirty years. She has three adult children and three grandchildren. She plays bocce, and enjoys swimming and long walks. She has given speeches at Alzheimer's walks for local groups in hope of changing the stigma of the diagnosis of Alzheimer's.

Jennifer Harrington works in the computer technology field and enjoys playing music, computer games, and movie night with her husband and four children. She cared for her mother through her journey with Alzheimer's disease and is now a volunteer for the Alzheimer's Association Northern California Chapter.

Karen Henley received her Bachelor of Arts degree in American Literature from Hofstra University in 1983. She continues to advocate for people with younger-onset Alzheimer's disease. Karen hopes to one day write a book documenting her family's journey with Alzheimer's.

Theresa Hettinger looks after her mom who has been struggling with Alzheimer's disease for many years. She sees firsthand the anguish of the Alzheimer's patient and their families. Theresa works in the non-profit sector and is also an advocate for pet adoptions, having rescued two dogs.

Marjorie Hilkert volunteers for the Alzheimer's Association Southeastern Virginia Chapter and serves on the Peninsula Alzheimer's Leadership Council. She is a certified trainer for the Memories in the Making Art program. With her mom living nearby, Marjorie and her husband John reside in Williamsburg, VA. E-mail her at marjoriehilkert@yahoo.com.

Julie Hornok has been married to her wonderful husband for sixteen years and is the mother of three children, including a daughter with autism. Julie enjoys writing about the constant (and sometimes painfully real) ups and downs of her family's journey through life with autism. E-mail her at julie_hornok@yahoo.com.

Dr. Steve Hume was diagnosed with Alzheimer's disease in May of 2007 at the age of sixty. Prior to his diagnosis, Dr. Hume was a clinician, consultant and senior manager in the behavioral health field for thirty-five years. He has a doctorate in clinical psychology and lives with his life partner, Candace, in Massachusetts. E-mail him at fbrap@aol.com.

Paul Hyckie is a Shiatsu therapist living in Toronto.

Jennie Ivey lives in Tennessee. She is the author of various works of fiction and nonfiction, including several stories in Chicken Soup for the Soul collections. Learn more at jennieivey.com.

Carrie Jackson began working in Alzheimer's care two years ago, as her father's battle with the disease was coming to an end. She is on the Alzheimer's Association Greater Illinois Chapter Junior Board, and is actively involved in fundraising, education, and advocacy. She also enjoys yoga, swimming, writing, music, and playing with her godson.

Joy Johnston is an experienced digital journalist. Her father's death from Alzheimer's complications in 2011 inspired her blog "The Memories Project", which was featured on NPR. Joy lives in Atlanta with her partner, two spoiled cats, and a goofy Pit Bull. E-mail her at joyjohnston.writer@gmail.com.

Laura Suihkonen Jones's husband Jay, diagnosed at fifty, was a member of the Alzheimer's Association Early-Stage Advisory Group. Laura received the Alzheimer's Association's Caregiver of the Year Award and Maureen Reagan Outstanding Advocate Award in 2011, and was a Soroptimist International Woman of Distinction in 2012.

Kitty Kennedy is a lifelong adventurer and storyteller. Her work with the Alzheimer's Association and her role as caregiver have opened new challenges and opportunities for learning.

Fred Kinsinger received a B.S. in engineering from Pennsylvania State University and an MBA from the University of Akron. He served as Captain in the U.S. Army during the Vietnam Era. After retiring as an engineering manager in the power generation business, he spent the next ten years managing his own technical sales company.

Doris Leddy is a breast cancer survivor, with two publications in *Coping with Cancer*. She was born in New York City. Doris has been an honored guest speaker at a breast cancer event, and she developed a cancer support group. Her passion for writing comes from personal true events in her life.

Cindy Legorreta clearly understands the value of starting over. She returned to college at fifty-five, getting married for the first time at sixty. She lives with her seafarer husband Ric in downtown New York. They are both excellent cooks; their lively household includes three cats and a beloved extended clan, two with Alzheimer's disease.

Mary Margaret Lehmann and Ken are grateful for the support and caring they have received from the Alzheimer's Association. Together, they are working for a world without Alzheimer's.

Tamera Leland received her Bachelors of Science in Nursing in 1997. She works as a Director of Nurses in a continuum of care facility for people with dementia. She has a son and a daughter-in-law, and will soon be blessed with her first grandchild!

Crescent LoMonaco used her knowledge from years working behind the chair and owning a hair salon to write the "Ask a Stylist" column for the *Santa Barbara Independent*. She is a frequent contributor to the

Chicken Soup for the Soul series. She lives on the California coast with her husband and son.

Joanne L. Lord is a Certified Clinical Research Coordinator at the University of Michigan. She has been conducting clinical trials and working with people who have Alzheimer's disease and related disorders and their families for over fifteen years. In her spare time she enjoys horseback riding, reading, photography, and martial arts.

James C. Magruder, an award-winning advertising copywriter and executive speechwriter, heads the marketing communications department at a Fortune 200 company. He's been published in *Writer's Digest*, *Writer's Journal*, *Marriage Partnership*, *HomeLife* and *Christian Communicator*. His blog about writing: www.thewritersrefuge. wordpress.com.

Mary Margaret Mann is an accomplished actress, author and speaker, specializing in one-woman performances. She brings alive to audiences her many characters ranging from Mary Lincoln to Elizabeth Barrett Browning to Mrs. Noah. She contributed to a book that is in the White House Library. Learn more at www.marymargaretmann.com.

Denise Marks is a freelance writer who strives to encourage and motivate others through writing and speaking. Her recently published children's book, *Remember the Rainbow*, was inspired by her three grandchildren. This is Denise's second contribution to the Chicken Soup for the Soul series. E-mail her at decemarks@chartermi.net.

Hank Mattimore was the director of the Sonoma County Alzheimer's Association for two years and the author of four books. He also served as a surrogate grandpa for five years at the intergenerational Children's Village in Sonoma County and is currently a commissioner on the Juvenile Justice Commission.

Jeri McBryde lives in a small southern town outside Memphis, TN.

She is retired and spends her days reading and working on her dream of publishing a novel. Jeri loves crocheting and chocolate. Her family and faith are the center of her life. This is her sixth story to appear in the Chicken Soup for the Soul series.

Joey McIntyre is a multi-talented international artist. In addition to being a member of the iconic group New Kids on the Block, Joey has sold more than 1 million solo albums worldwide. As a singer, songwriter, actor and Broadway performer, his passion continues to fuel his acclaimed entertainment pursuits.

Amy Merrill is a seventeen-year-old high school senior, a competitive cheerleader, and year-round soccer player. This short story is dedicated to her grandfather, Lewis Russell Darling, because it is the best way to show the world how much she loved him.

Carolyn Mers lives in the metro St. Louis area with her husband, Dan. They have three grown daughters and two grandsons. Carolyn began journaling during the first ten years of her mother's dementia process, which eventually became her first book, *The Alzheimer's Roller Coaster, The Story of Our Ride.*

Sandy Morris is a full-time caregiver to her husband with Alzheimer's way too early in life. She is a mom to her two sports-minded teens and continues to work full-time as a special education teacher. She survives on coffee, prayer and the support of family and friends. She blogs through the chaos, and strives to find joy in the storm of life.

Ann Napoletan is a freelance writer, blogger, passionate advocate, and former caregiver to her mother. She is committed to fighting Alzheimer's and other forms of dementia and helping caregivers navigate their own unique journeys. Ann is also active with USAgainstAlzheimer's and the Alzheimer's Association.

Evangeline Neve lived in many places before settling in Nepal in

1996, where she works with underprivileged children and writes about travel, food, family and cats. When not busy, you can find her at home with a good book and one of her cats on her lap. Learn more at www.evangelineneve.com.

Robert S. Nussbaum is an attorney by day and a writer in the very early morning hours. This is his fifth story published in the Chicken Soup for the Soul series. In addition, more than thirty of his letters have been published in *The New York Times*.

Linda O'Connell, an accomplished writer and teacher from St. Louis, MO, treasures every moment with her family. A positive thinker, she writes from the heart, bares her soul, and finds humor in everyday situations. Linda enjoys a hearty laugh, dark chocolate and walks on the beach. Contact her at http://lindaoconnell.blogspot.com.

Dale Adams O'Neill is a vice president and former English instructor in a North Carolina Community College. She enjoys volunteering with the Alzheimer's Association. She is especially grateful for God's gift of her granddaughter, Addyson, whose love helped her through the sorrow of losing her mother to Alzheimer's.

Rhonda Penders is a published author living in upstate New York. Her father, Bill Mosher, suffered from dementia for seven years before passing away in September 2013. Her romance novels, published under the pen name Roni Adams, can be found for sale at www.thewildrosepress.com.

Wendy Poole feels honored to have this story published. The book will be a wonderful/comforting/inspirational resource for so many. Wendy continues to teach part-time at a community college in Toronto. When not traveling or spending time with friends and family, she also enjoys writing stories about her grandchildren.

Sarah Rafferty currently plays Donna Paulsen on USA Network's hit series *Suits*. She has appeared on numerous TV shows and in many professional theatre productions. Sarah splits her time between Los Angeles and Toronto with her husband and two daughters.

Johanna Richardson lost her mother, stepdad, mother-in-law and grandmother-in-law to dementia. She received her master's degree from the University of San Francisco. Johanna adores being with her husband and family. She loves reading, music, film, traveling and serving as Peer Volunteer for the national Alzheimer's Association.

Lisa R. Richardson holds a B.A. degree in Public Relations and is currently pursuing a master's degree in Human Resource Development. She lives in Georgetown, KY, and writes stories to honor the memory of the West sisters, all of whom have suffered from Alzheimer's disease.

Dr. Kelle Z. Riley, author, scientist and safety/martial arts expert, has been featured in forums from local newspapers to national television. Her debut novel, *Dangerous Affairs*, was praised for accurately highlighting women's issues in an easily accessible, entertaining format. Learn more at www.kellezriley.net.

Sioux Roslawski's father, Ollie Kortjohn, and her family friend, Jim Gannaway, died after long battles with Alzheimer's. Sioux is a freelance writer and a third grade teacher. For her, writing about her loved ones is a way to keep them with her... forever. Learn more at http://siouxspage.blogspot.com.

Amy Sayers works as an instructional coach, partnering with teachers to find ways to bring technology into the classroom in meaningful ways. Along with teaching, Amy also enjoys teaching childbirth education classes, as well as working at Notre Dame Stadium as captain of the east sideline.

Laurie Rueter Schultz received her BSEd and her MA in English.

She lives in O'Fallon with her husband Kevin and their two children, Adison and Brody. Their third child is expected in June. Laurie teaches English at Marquette High School in Chesterfield, MO. This story is for her mom.

Sherry Sharp lives in Richmond, VA with her husband Richard, two Golden Retrievers, Daisy and Gabby, and Tibetan Spaniel Reesey. She is the mother of two daughters, two sons-in-law and four grandchildren. Sherry enjoys writing Christian devotions, hand quilting, spending time with her family and playing with her four-legged friends.

Deborah Shouse is a writer, speaker, editor and creativity catalyst. Her writing has appeared in *The Washington Post*, *The Christian Science Monitor*, *Reader's Digest*, *Newsweek*, *Woman's Day* and *Family Circle*. She wrote *Love in the Land of Dementia: Finding Hope in the Caregiver's Journey*. Read more at www.deborahshousewrites.wordpress.com.

Ann Marie Skerl was a nurse for thirty-five years. She retired after being diagnosed with younger-onset, early-stage Alzheimer's disease at fifty-five. She attends an Alzheimer's support group and is active in advocating for Alzheimer's awareness. She also enjoys spending time with her children and grandchildren.

A former businessman, **Reverend Jim Solomon** has helped over 1,000 families and individuals across the nation experience life-change through counsel and care. He lives with his wife and two children in Newtown, CT, serving as Pastor of New Hope Community Church and chaplain of the Newtown Police Department.

Sara Spaulding is the daughter of a West Point graduate and has traveled around the U.S. and Europe. She received her master of technical communication from Colorado State University. She enjoys skiing, scuba diving, hiking, mountain and road biking, and treasures time with family, friends and her Border Collies.

Julie Staffen is an award-winning children's author from Michigan. She is the writer of the children's series, Krista Kay Adventures, which she is completing while working on a new series for boys. In her spare time Julie enjoys travel and time with her husband and son.

Bern Nadette Stanis is best known for her role as Thelma Evans in the groundbreaking sitcom *Good Times*. She travels the world as the author of three books. Her most recent work, *The Last Night: A Caregiver's Journey*, profiles a loving daughter and her mother's Alzheimer's diagnosis.

Amy L. Stout is a wife, mommy, and autism advocate who loves travel, coffee houses, books and especially Jesus! As a child of the King, her tiara is often missing, dusty, bent out of shape, or crooked, but she will always be his treasured princess. Contact her at histreasuredprincess.blogspot.com or Brightencorner@hotmail.com.

Nancy Sturm taught English for twenty-one years and taught and co-directed the South Central Kansas Writing Project. She supervises student teachers for Wichita State University. Nancy enjoys volunteering at church, walking on nature trails, learning to tap dance, and writing a devotional blog.

K. Thorp is currently enrolled in college at SUNY Cortland. She hopes to soon be accepted into the New Media Design program. She plans to be a graphic designer or a photographer someday. Her hobbies include photography, painting, drawing, cooking, and baking.

Pat Tomlinson, the fourth of six children, is a mother, proud grandmother, aunt to several nieces and nephews, and a grateful friend to many. She continues to entertain audiences with the storytelling skills honed from her teaching career. Many thanks to Caryl, Debbie, and Lyn for their inspiration and encouragement.

Susie Van Den Ameele, a longtime resident of Seattle, WA, works in the biotech industry. She loves trail racing and hiking the beautiful Pacific Northwest with her daughter Addy, appreciating the little things in life on the trails. She has revived her interest in dress designing and loves watching Addy find creative outlets of her own.

Jennifer Waggener works for the Alzheimer's Association West Virginia Chapter. She and her husband enjoy adventures in travel and are quite infatuated with learning the fine art of excellent grandparenting under the careful guidance of their first grandchild, Henley.

Samantha Ducloux Waltz is an award-winning freelance writer and caregiver for her husband who has Alzheimer's. Her personal essays can be seen in Chicken Soup for the Soul and other anthologies. She has also written under the name Samellyn Wood. Learn more at www.pathsofthought.com.

Sue Watkins, caregiver for her husband Lew, holds college degrees and credentials in Health Information Management and Cancer Surveillance. Previous writing experiences include professional textbook and peer journals. She enjoys reading, quilting, playing golf and travel, particularly with her husband. E-mail her at watkinssue1@gmail.com.

Richard Weinman, Emeritus Professor at Oregon State University, knows Alzheimer's well: his wife, Ginny, seventy-seven, mother of the couple's twelve children, died in December, after fifteen years with the disease. Their life together is visited in Richard's memoir, *Two Different Worlds*.

John White graduated from Harding College in 1968, is a Vietnam veteran and has worked as a long-term care administrator since 1976. John continues to serve seniors today, has been married for forty-five years, is a high school umpire in Alabama, plays baseball in national tournaments and enjoys his four grandchildren.

Susan DeWitt Wilder lives in Scarborough, ME, and in Davis, NC with her husband Paul Austin and her perspicacious Welsh Corgi, Pattie. Since her essay was written, Susan's father has died and her mother, always good-natured, now lives happily in a nearby assisted living facility. E-mail her at swilder@gwi.net.

Bruce Michael Williams is a mechanical/biomedical engineer. His hobbies include building airplanes, flying, cooking and now, writing. He resides at Spruce Creek Fly-In with his lovely wife and Cleco the Labradoodle, where he continues writing. He has started a support group for caregivers. E-mail him at gasketguy1@gmail.com.

Sue Young is a transplanted Brit who has lived in the U.S. since 1978. Her hobbies are photography, travel, animals and reading. She works full-time and writes whenever she has a spare moment.

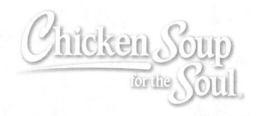

Meet Our Authors

Amy Newmark has been Chicken Soup for the Soul's publisher, coauthor, and editor-in-chief for the last six years, after a 30-year career as a writer, speaker, financial analyst, and business executive in the worlds of finance and telecommunications. Amy is a Chartered Financial Analyst and a *magna cum laude* graduate of Harvard College, where she majored in Portuguese, minored in French, and traveled extensively. She and her husband have four grown children.

After a long career writing books on telecommunications, voluminous financial reports, business plans, and corporate press releases, Chicken Soup for the Soul is a breath of fresh air for Amy. She loves creating these life-changing books for Chicken Soup for the Soul's wonderful readers. She has coauthored and/or edited more than 100 Chicken Soup for the Soul books.

You can reach Amy with any questions or comments through webmaster@chickensoupforthesoul.com and you can follow her on Twitter @amynewmark or @chickensoupsoul.

Angela Timashenka Geiger is the Chief Strategy Officer for the Alzheimer's Association based in Chicago.

As a member of the senior management team, Geiger works day-to-day across all divisions to coordinate and execute strategy. She has accountability for more than $225 million in annual fundraising, programs and services reaching over 1 million people per year, brand/marketing, corporate initiatives, and diversity.

Geiger has successfully led Association efforts to develop and expand programmatic offerings, marketing and fundraising to increase concern and awareness, maximize impact in the fight against Alzheimer's disease, and improve the lives of those affected. She organized an integrated consumer education campaign to raise concern about Alzheimer's, which featured the Association's first nationwide paid ads, public relations outreach and grassroots outreach by chapters. She spearheaded the launch of a series of Early-Stage Town Halls across the nation as a platform for people living in the early stages of Alzheimer's to discuss issues and share helpful resources, programs and services. Additionally, her leadership significantly expanded the reach and impact of the signature awareness and fundraising event for the organization, the rebranded Alzheimer's Association Walk to End Alzheimer's®. Walk began with nine chapters raising $149,000 in 1989 and has grown to raise more than $57 million in 2013. Since the event's inception, Walk has raised more than $546 million.

Geiger has significant experience in strategic marketing and program development for nonprofits. Prior to joining the Alzheimer's Association, she spent eight years at the American Cancer Society (ACS) in a variety of leadership roles and also worked for the American Lung Association and for higher education institutions.

She has her B.A. and MBA from the University of Pittsburgh and has contributed to a variety of conferences and publications, including *The Shriver Report: A Woman's Nation Takes on Alzheimer's*.

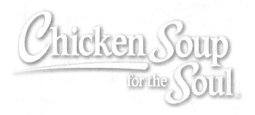

Thank You

We owe huge thanks to all of the people who submitted stories for this book. We know that you poured your hearts and souls into the thousands of stories and poems that you shared with us, and ultimately with other families affected by Alzheimer's and other dementias. As we read and edited these stories, we were truly amazed by your strength, your honesty, and your great advice. We appreciate your willingness to share these inspiring and revealing stories with our readers. You are helping millions of people.

We could only publish a small percentage of the stories that were submitted, but we read every single one and even the ones that do not appear in the book had an influence on us and on the final manuscript. We owe special thanks to Brett Armstrong, Senior Associate Director, Editorial & Creative Content at the Alzheimer's Association, who read all the submissions to this volume, and narrowed down the list to a manageable size. She is a great editor. Chicken Soup for the Soul senior editor Barbara LoMonaco, who lost her own mother to Alzheimer's, read all the stories as well, and managed the entire process of story selection with a large group of people at the Association who worked on this book in addition to Brett, including Kate Meyer, Monica Moreno, and Jenny Maxse. Thanks also to the staff at the Association who helped promote and collect submissions, including Mary Beth Lantzy, David Lusk, and Emily Shubeck. We are also grateful to Ingrid Wells, who managed the partnership aspects of the project for the Association.

Chicken Soup for the Soul's VP and assistant publisher D'ette Corona did her normal masterful job of working with the contributors to approve our edits and answer any questions we had. And managing editor and production coordinator Kristiana Pastir proofread and managed the metamorphosis from Word document to printed book.

We also owe a special thanks to creative director and book producer, Brian Taylor at Pneuma Books, for his brilliant vision for the cover and the interior.

~Amy and Angela

alzheimer's ⊕ association®

About the Alzheimer's Association

The Alzheimer's Association is the world's leading voluntary health organization in Alzheimer's care, support and research. Founded in 1980 by a group of family caregivers and individuals interested in research, the Association includes the national office in Chicago, the public policy office in Washington, D.C., and chapters in communities nationwide.

Currently, at least 44 million people worldwide are living with dementia. In the United States alone, more than 5 million have Alzheimer's, and over 15 million are serving as their caregivers. The Alzheimer's Association addresses this global epidemic by providing education and support to the millions who face dementia every day, while advancing critical research toward methods of treatment, prevention and, ultimately, a cure.

We provide care and support to those affected.
- The Alzheimer's Association 24/7 Helpline (800-272-3900) is available all day, every day.
- Our award-winning website at alz.org® is a rich resource that includes information for people living in the early stage of the disease (alz.org/IHaveAlz) and caregivers (alz.org/care).
- Chapters host thousands of support groups and educational sessions annually. Find a chapter near you at alz.org/findus.

We accelerate research across the globe.

- We are the largest nonprofit funder of Alzheimer's research. Since 1982, our International Research Grant Program has committed over $315 million to more than 2,200 best-of-field grant proposals, leading to exciting advances including the development of Pittsburgh Compound B (PIB), the first radiotracer capable of showing beta-amyloid in the living brain during a PET scan.

- The Alzheimer's Association International Conference® (AAIC®) is the world's largest conference of its kind, bringing researchers together to report on groundbreaking studies. The conference has served as a platform for major milestones in Alzheimer's research, including the release of new diagnostic criteria.

- We lead the World Wide Alzheimer's Disease Neuroimaging Initiative (WW-ADNI), a consortium of international Alzheimer's investigators. The sharing of ADNI data across the globe has demonstrated a significant return on investment, enabling researchers who were not funded to participate in scientific progress.

We advocate for the needs and rights of people facing Alzheimer's.

- The Association has helped pass landmark legislation, including the National Alzheimer's Project Act, which mandated a national plan to fight Alzheimer's disease. The National Alzheimer's Plan addresses the escalating Alzheimer's crisis and coordinates efforts across the federal government.

- We call for an increased commitment to Alzheimer's funding from the federal government. In 2014, the Association helped secure a $122 million increase for Alzheimer's research, education, outreach and caregiver support.

- We demand better access to diagnosis and care planning so those with Alzheimer's can receive the best treatments and plan for the future.

We're here all day, every day.
Call 800-272-3900 or visit alz.org.

- Connect with a chapter. Participate in a support group, attend an educational workshop or volunteer.
- Advocate for those affected and urge legislators to make Alzheimer's a national priority.
- Participate in Walk to End Alzheimer's®, the world's largest event to raise awareness and funds for Alzheimer's care, support and research.
- Donate to advance vital research and further care and support programs.

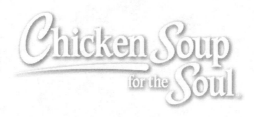

Sharing Happiness, Inspiration, and Wellness

Real people sharing real stories, every day, all over the world. In 2007, *USA Today* named *Chicken Soup for the Soul* one of the five most memorable books in the last quarter-century. With over 100 million books sold to date in the U.S. and Canada alone, more than 200 titles in print, and translations into more than 40 languages, "chicken soup for the soul" is one of the world's best-known phrases.

Today, 20 years after we first began sharing happiness, inspiration and wellness through our books, we continue to delight our readers with new titles, but have also evolved beyond the bookstore, with wholesome and balanced pet food, delicious nutritious comfort food, and a major motion picture in development. Whatever you're doing, wherever you are, Chicken Soup for the Soul is "always there for you™." Thanks for reading!